KT-492-105

WITHDRAWN

04596117

MODERN
Flexitarian

MODERN
Flexitarian

VEG-BASED RECIPES YOU CAN FLEX TO ADD FISH, MEAT, OR DAIRY

Contents

Burgers, Tacos, and Wraps

Beginning a Flexitarian Diet

Getting started is easier than you may think. These simple tips will help with your first steps into flexitarianism, with nutritional information to ensure you're eating a balanced diet as well as storecupboard suggestions and an example meal plan to make cooking easier.

What is a flexitarian diet?

"Flexitarian" was coined more than 20 years ago to refer to people who are predominantly vegetarian, but occasionally include meat or fish in their diet. For that reason, a flexitarian diet can also be referred to as a "semi-vegetarian" diet. More recently, as people are becoming increasingly aware of the benefits of a completely plant-based diet, a number of flexitarians also consciously reduce their intake of other animal products, such as dairy and eggs.

Flexitarianism is a lifestyle choice, not another temporary fad diet. People's motivations for adopting a flexitarian diet differ (see p12), but generally relate to their health or to a concern for animal welfare or the environment.

A flexitarian diet is about so much more than just omitting the meat from your meals; it's about making smarter food choices in general. Emphasising good quality, minimally processed foods from sustainable sources – which are not only better for your health but for the environment too – increases the nutrient density of your diet, thereby boosting your intake of essential vitamins, minerals, and beneficial phytochemicals from plant-based foods.

Starting a flexitarian diet is exciting and will introduce you to a whole range of plant-based alternatives to meat, including beans, lentils, and soy products (such as tofu and tempeh). Therefore, rather than seeing a flexitarian diet as restrictive or limiting, view it as an opportunity to expand your culinary horizons to a new world of delicious dishes that you and your family will love.

A common question people ask is about the amount of meat considered appropriate to include in a flexitarian diet. The great thing about this diet is the lack of rules – it's entirely up to you how often you choose to include meals with meat in your diet. To reap the maximum health benefits, you would ideally want to aim to reduce your meat intake to one serving per week, but the only commitments you need to make to call yourself a flexitarian is to consciously reduce your meat intake and to embrace more plant-based meals.

A flexitarian diet includes:
- Dairy products, such as cow's milk, yogurt, and cheese*
- Eggs*
- Legumes (pulses), such as chickpeas and lentils
- Vegetables
- Fruits
- Nuts and seeds
- Wholegrains and their products, such as brown rice, pasta, and bread

*People who follow a flexitarian diet may also choose to reduce their intake of dairy and eggs.

A flexitarian diet occasionally includes:
- Red meats, such as beef and lamb
- Poultry, such as chicken and turkey
- Fish and seafood, such as salmon, tuna, and prawns

A flexitarian diet minimises:
- Processed meats, including bacon, salami, and ham
- Refined grains, such as white rice
- Refined grain products, such as white bread, biscuits, and cakes
- Added sugars, particularly white sugar
- Fast foods, particularly fried foods such as chips
- Processed snack foods, such as crisps

Why go flexitarian?

One of the best things about flexitarianism is that it is not a stressful lifestyle change. As a flexitarian, you can pick and choose when to eat only plant-based foods, or when to add animal products, as it suits you. Additionally, every time you do enjoy a plant-based meal, you're making a positive contribution to your health and the environment, as well as reducing the negative impact of your food choices on animals. It can also be cheaper, too!

Health benefits

Many flexitarian staple foods are packed with dietary fibre, which help keep the digestive system healthy. Unprocessed plant-based foods including fruits, vegetables, wholegrains, legumes, nuts, and seeds, are all good sources of both soluble and insoluble dietary fibre, while prebiotic fibre (which promotes the growth of beneficial bacteria in the gut) can be found in pulses such as chickpeas and lentils, wholegrains such as barley and rye, and a diverse range of vegetables such as onions, garlic, artichokes, and asparagus. Animal products, on the other hand, contain very little dietary fibre.

By being flexitarian and eating a balanced amount of meat, you may also help to reduce your chances of developing certain cancers. The World Health Organization (WHO) has classified red meat as a Group 2A carcinogen, meaning that there is enough evidence to suggest that it probably causes cancer of the bowel and colon, while processed meats (such as hot dogs and salami) are classified as a Group 1 carcinogen, which means there is convincing evidence that they cause cancer. Meanwhile, large population studies have shown that predominantly plant-based diets – including semi-vegetarian diets – are associated with a lower risk of developing colorectal cancer.

In addition, diets rich in fruits and vegetables, wholegrains, legumes, and nuts are consistently associated with a lower risk of developing type 2 diabetes. By limiting your red meat and poultry intake and instead choosing plant-based meals made up of legumes, vegetables, and wholegrains, you'll reduce your risk of developing type 2 diabetes.

Environmental benefits

Our current global food production system is the single largest driver of environmental degradation, contributing to climate change, biodiversity loss, and unsustainable land and water use. To conserve the health of the planet while feeding a growing global population that is projected to reach 10 billion people by 2050, a team of scientists from the EAT-Lancet Commission – an organisation of 37 diet and food sustainability experts – have called for a global shift to a flexitarian-style "planetary health diet". This diet consists of fruits, vegetables, wholegrains, nuts, seeds, plant proteins (including beans and lentils), and unsaturated plant oils; it includes only modest amounts of meat and dairy.

Cost benefits

Whether you are moving to a flexitarian, vegetarian, or vegan diet, there are hidden costs that can develop, especially if you're relying on ready meals and processed foods. But this doesn't need to be the case. In fact, being flexitarian is arguably much cheaper than regularly eating meat or fish, as these are the most expensive items on a standard shopping list. Expensive convenience items – such as faux meats – can be easily avoided by learning how to prepare pulses and tofu so that they're appealing and delicious. Before you know it, you will have a pantry full of canned or dried pulses, wholegrains, nuts and seeds, as well as fresh fruits and vegetables, that you can rely on to build weekly meals on a budget.

Animal welfare benefits

The production of meat, dairy, or eggs is a business and, like any other, it must be profitable in order to survive. Animal welfare concerns can often be sacrificed in order to keep costs for consumers down, which for many people is a key reason why they choose to reduce their intake of animal products. If and when you do buy meat, fish, and eggs, look for organic certification, which should be an indicator of good quality and higher welfare standards.

How to be flexitarian

As the word suggests, the great thing about flexitarianism is its flexibility. If you're trying to go flexitarian for the first time, you have the freedom to make as many or as few changes as you feel comfortable with, and take it from there. Here are some tips and inspiration to help you get started and to stay on track.

- Start small. Commit to just one meat-free day per week, such as "Meat Free Monday", and steadily adjust your diet from there.

- If you're finding it tricky to adjust from the traditional "meat and two veg" idea of mealtimes, make the most of meat-alternative products. Supermarkets now stock a wide selection of vegetarian and vegan options that have a similar taste and texture to meat, including burgers, sausages, and faux chicken fillets and nuggets. While they aren't as nutrient-rich as unprocessed wholefoods like beans and lentils, they're a great option when you're adjusting to meat-free meals.

- Instead of cutting meat from your meals entirely, try substituting half the meat content for a plant-based source of protein, such as beans or lentils. For instance, you could bulk up your spaghetti Bolognese with brown lentils, which will boost the fibre and phytochemical content of the dish significantly. This fifty–fifty approach allows you to halve your red meat intake while still enjoying the flavour and textures you love.

- If you feel held back by your cooking skills or are stuck for ideas, seek out a local vegetarian or vegan cooking class to boost your kitchen confidence. You could also visit a local vegan restaurant to familiarise yourself with the range of tastes and textures plant-based cooking can offer. Try a few dishes, then have a go at recreating them at home.

- Include your friends and family in your new diet by hosting a plant-based dinner. Who knows? You might inspire them to go flexitarian, too.

- Take inspiration from cuisines that traditionally use beans and lentils, and bring out their flavour with herbs and spices. Try a hearty Mediterranean soup or stew that uses beans, an Indian dhal or curry with lentils, peas or chickpeas, or a Mexican chilli that makes the most of kidney or pinto beans.

- Prepare large batches of your favourite plant-based recipes, then freeze the leftovers or save them for lunch the following day. That way, if you're short on time, you won't get caught out without a flexitarian option to hand.

- Sit down on a Sunday and plan the week of meals ahead. This will help you to save time and money, and to minimise food waste. See pages 26–27 for an example weekly meal plan.

A balanced flexitarian diet

When making any dietary change, it's important to be aware of how it will impact your day-to-day nutritional intake. For example, if you decide to omit dairy products from your diet, you need to make sure you're still meeting your body's needs for key nutrients that dairy once provided, such as calcium, iodine, and vitamin B12. If you think you may benefit from one-on-one dietary advice, speak to a dietician or GP, who will be able to help you plan your new diet to ensure you are meeting your personal nutritional needs.

The five food groups

Outlined below and opposite are five food groups that each provide similar amounts of key nutrients per serving. The foods listed within these groups will make up the core of your flexitarian diet. While it is important that you are including the recommended number of servings from the five food groups each day, you should also try to include a variety of foods from within each group, as different foods within the same groups differ in their nutrient content. There is an endless number of delicious meals you can create by combining foods from all the food groups. By doing so, you'll be able to make healthy food choices effortlessly, as these whole and minimally processed foods retain most of their original nutritional content.

The information given here is based on an average adult diet. The recommended daily number of servings of each food group will differ for toddlers, children, teenagers, and those who are pregant or breastfeeding. Consult the NHS Eat Well website for the most accurate advice.

Servings per day

Adults 5–6

Vegetables and legumes

You can't eat too many vegetables! Vegetables, legumes and beans are a good source of folate, fibre, vitamin C, potassium, and magnesium. They also provide a range of beneficial phytochemicals, so try to eat a varied and colourful range of vegetables each day.

1 serving, containing around 100–350kJ, is roughly equal to:

- 75g (2½oz) cooked vegetables such as broccoli, corn, spinach, pumpkin or carrots
- 75g (2½oz) cooked dried or canned beans, peas, or lentils
- 75g (2½oz) green leafy or raw salad vegetables
- ½ medium potato or other starchy vegetables, such as sweet potato
- 1 medium tomato

Fruit

A serving of fruit provides a good source of folate, dietary fibre, vitamin C, provitamin A carotenoids, potassium, and magnesium. Some fruits can also contain a range of beneficial phytochemicals, such as the antioxidants found in berries.

1 serving, containing around 350kJ, is roughly equal to:

- 1 medium piece of fruit, such as an apple, orange, or banana
- 2 small pieces of fruit, such as kiwi fruits, plums, or apricots
- 150g (5½oz) diced fruit, such as pineapple or mango (including fruit canned in natural juice)

A 30g (1oz) portion of dried fruit, such as sultanas or dried apricots, or 120ml (4fl oz) of fruit juice (with no added sugar) can also count as one serve of fruit, but only occasionally as these choices can increase the risk of tooth decay.

Adults 2

Servings per day

Adults 3–6

Starchy, grain-based foods

Starchy foods should make up just over a third of every meal you eat, as they help satisfy your hunger and are a good source of carbohydrates, protein, dietary fibre, magnesium, B vitamins, vitamin E, phosphorous, iron, and zinc. It's important to choose wholegrain or wholemeal foods wherever possible, rather than highly refined and processed varieties, such as white bread. Refined grains have been stripped of germ and bran layers, which significantly reduces their vitamin, mineral, and antioxidant content.

1 serving, containing around 500kJ, is roughly equal to:

- 1 slice (40g/1½oz) bread
- ½ medium (40g/1½oz) bread roll or flatbread
- 75–120g (2½–4¼oz) cooked rice or other grains, such as pasta, noodles, cous cous, polenta or semolina
- 120g (4¼oz) cooked porridge
- 30g (1oz) wheat cereal flakes
- 30g (1oz) muesli or rolled oats

Adults 2–3

Lean meat, poultry, fish, eggs, nuts, seeds and legumes

On a flexitarian diet, you'll automatically be eating less meat, poultry, fish, and eggs. Luckily, the plant-based options in this food group also provide a good source of protein, iron, and zinc. However, while meat, fish, and eggs are all good sources of vitamin B12, the plant foods in this group are not. See page 20 for more information about vitamin B12 to ensure you're getting the right amount on a flexitarian diet.

1 serving, containing around 500–600kJ, is roughly equal to:

- 65g (2⅛oz) cooked lean red meat (90–100g/3¼–3½oz raw)
- 80g (2¾oz) cooked poultry (100g/3½oz raw)
- 100g (3½oz) cooked fish (115g/4oz raw) or 1 small can of fish
- 2 large (120g/4½oz) eggs
- 150g (5½oz) cooked legumes (dried or canned)
- 170g (6oz) firm tofu
- 30g (1oz) nuts or seeds, or their pastes or butters (only occasionally as they provide fewer nutrients)

Experts recommend that you eat no more than 7 servings of red meat per week. This shouldn't be too much of an issue on a flexitarian diet, as you'll already be aiming to cut back on red meat.

Milk, yogurt, cheese and their alternatives

This food group contains a variety of dairy and non-dairy options, which caters perfectly to a flexitarian diet. Milk, yogurt, cheese, and their alternatives are a good source of protein and calcium. While dairy products are also an important source of the mineral iodine, dairy alternatives – such as soy milk and tofu – are not. See page 21 for more information about iodine.

1 serving, containing around 500–600kJ, is rougly equal to:

- 250ml (9fl oz) cow's or calcium-fortified non-dairy milk
- 40g (1½oz) hard cheese
- 120g (4¼oz) soft cheese, such as ricotta
- 200g (7oz) yogurt
- 100g (3½oz) calcium-set firm tofu (check ingredients for calcium sulphate E516 or calcium chloride E509)
- 60g (2oz) canned sardines
- 100g (3½oz) canned pink salmon with bones

It is recommended you choose reduced-fat varieties of milk, yogurt, and soft cheese, and keep your hard cheese intake to around two or three serves per week. Keep in mind that reduced-fat varieties of dairy products are not suitable for children under the age of two due to their high energy needs for growth. Infants (aged under 12 months) should not be given cow's milk as a main drink; breastmilk or formula is recommended as the main source of milk.

Adults 2.5–4

"Sometimes" foods

You may wonder where cake, pastries, ice cream, chocolate, crisps, alcohol, and other processed and fast foods sit within these five food groups. The straight answer is that they don't. These are discretionary foods, and are not necessary for a healthy diet because they don't provide important nutrients. That being said, occasionally including these foods in your diet – in small amounts – doesn't pose a risk to health. A good way to think of these foods is as "sometimes" foods.

Macronutrients

Protein, carbohydrates, and fat are the three main macronutrients that the body needs in large amounts to provide it with energy. When adopting a flexitarian diet, you may be worried about getting enough protein because you'll be reducing your intake of meat, fish, and eggs (which are commonly thought of as "protein" foods) and increasing your intake of foods such as beans and lentils (which are commonly considered (carbohydrates). Unfortunately, this view is overly simplistic, as most wholefoods – unlike those that are highly processed – actually provide a combination of protein, carbohydrates, and fat. For example, two slices of a good-quality wholegrain bread, often considered to be purely a source of carbohydrates, actually provide 11 grams of protein and 5 grams of fat, as well as 19 grams of carbohydrate.

Carbohydrates

Our bodies obtain energy in the form of glucose from carbohydrates. Glucose fuels our body's cells, powering our brain and muscles. Carbohydrates are predominantly found in plant foods, with the exception of the sugar lactose, which is found in dairy products. Below are foods with good sources of carbohydrates to include daily in your flexitarian diet.

- Fruits, such as bananas, apples and berries
- Vegetables, particularly starchy vegetables such as potatoes, sweet potatoes, and sweetcorn
- Wholegrains, including brown rice, quinoa and oats, and wholegrain products, such as bread, pasta and noodles
- Pulses, including beans, peas, chickpeas and lentils

Protein

This vital macronutrient is important for tissue building and repair, growth and maintenance of muscle mass, and the maintenance of healthy, strong bones. Protein is made up of twenty amino acids, nine of which are essential, which means that they can't be made by the body and must be obtained through the diet. The foods listed below are all good sources of protein, and contain all nine essential amino acids, for you to include in your daily diet.

Animal foods

- 65g (2⅛oz) cooked lean meat, such as lean beef, lamb, or pork (provides 20–22g of protein)
- 80g (2¾oz) cooked poultry, such as skinless grilled chicken breast (provides 24g of protein)
- 100g (3½oz) cooked white or oily fish, such as salmon or whiting (provides 22–24g of protein)
- 2 large eggs (provides 12g of protein)

Plant foods

- 170g (6oz) firm tofu (provides 20g of protein)
- 100g (3½oz) tempeh (provides 18g of protein)
- 150g (5½oz) cooked legumes, such as beans, peas, chickpeas, and lentils (provides 10–12g of protein)

If you choose to omit fish from your diet, plant-derived omega-3 supplements are available, made from microalgae.

Fats

A certain amount of fat is essential for the body to function; it is a concentrated source of energy and it aids the absorption of fat-soluble nutrients, including vitamins A and E. There are two main types of dietary fats: saturated and unsaturated. Saturated fats – found mostly in animal products – are associated with negative health effects, and so should be limited. The beauty of a flexitarian diet is that by reducing your meat intake, you'll be reducing your intake of saturated fat, not to mention cholesterol. The healthier unsaturated fats play an important part in a flexitarian diet and are associated with health benefits. Below are some good sources of these healthy unsaturated fats, but keep in mind that unless you have high energy needs or need to gain weight, your body doesn't need an overly large amount of fats, even the healthy ones.

- Nuts and seeds, such as sunflower seeds, pumpkin seeds, almonds and walnuts
- Wholegrains, such as rolled oats
- Soy products, including tofu, tempeh, and soy milk
- Oily fish, such as salmon
- Avocados
- Olive oil and other vegetable oils

It is also important to ensure that your diet includes good sources of the essential omega-3 fatty acids ALA, EPA, and DHA. ALA is found in good amounts in walnuts, chia seeds, and flaxseeds, whereas oily fish is the richest dietary source of EPA and DHA.

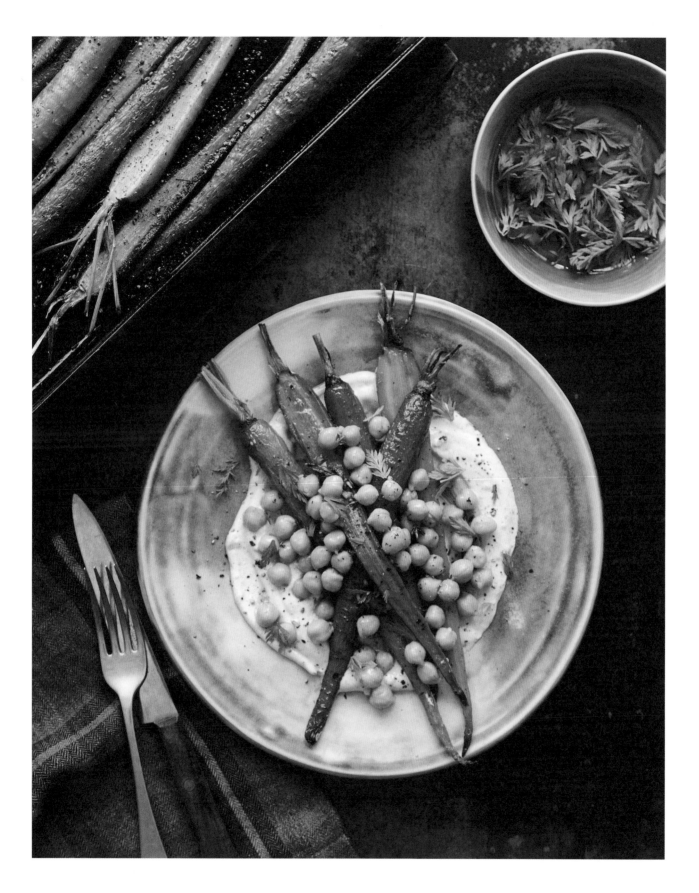

Vitamins

We are unable to synthesise vitamins in our body and so must obtain these essential nutrients – needed only in small amounts – through our diet. On a flexitarian diet, it's important to make sure you're paying attention to the following vitamins, which can fall short when your meat and dairy intakes are reduced.

Vitamin A
Important for vision, healthy skin, iron metabolism, and immune-system function, vitamin A has two types: preformed vitamin A, which is primarily found in dairy products, and provitamin A, which exists in many vegetables as carotenoids that our bodies are able to convert to the active form of vitamin A. Vegetables rich in provitamin A carotenoids include carrots, sweet potatoes, pumpkins, kale, spinach, and red peppers.

Vitamin D
Foods such as oily fish, eggs, and fortified milks do contain some vitamin D, but the majority of vitamin D required by the body is derived from safe sun exposure. Depending on where you live, it might be a good idea to take a vitamin D supplement through the cooler months of the year, when UV levels are low. Speak to your GP or a dietitian for more information about an appropriate supplement for you.

Vitamin B12
Our bodies receive the important vitamin B12 from animal foods in our diet. Vitamin B12 is required for cell division, blood formation, neurological structure and function, energy metabolism, psychological function, and immunity. Because plant foods don't contain vitamin B12, if you've reduced your meat and dairy intake you may need to take a vitamin B12 supplement to ensure you're meeting your body's daily requirement. Certain brands of speciality foods such as soy milk and vegetarian sausages are fortified with the vitamin, meaning it has been added by the manufacturer. However, three servings of these fortified foods are required every day in order to meet the body's needs. Speak to your GP or a dietitian for more information.

Minerals

Like vitamins, minerals are must-have nutrients which we are unable to synthesise in our body and must obtain through our diet. They are inorganic elements which are classified into two groups: major minerals which are required in larger amounts, such as calcium and otassium, and trace elements which are required in smaller amounts, such as iron and zinc. By eating a balanced flexitarian diet, you can easily meet your body's mineral requirements, but it's worth making sure you eat good sources of calcium, iron, zinc, and iodine.

Calcium
This mineral is essential for nerve and muscle function, blood coagulation, energy metabolism and to keep bones and teeth healthy and strong. It is most commonly known to be sourced from dairy products, but there are plenty of plant-based sources for those who wish to reduce their daily consumption.

Animal foods that contain calcium

- 250ml (9fl oz) cow's milk (provides 320mg of calcium)
- 200g (7oz) natural yogurt (provides 340mg of calcium)
- 40g (½oz) hard cheese (provides 320mg of calcium)
- 100g (3½oz) canned pink salmon (provides 190mg of calcium)

Plant foods that contain calcium

- 250ml (9fl oz) calcium-fortified non-dairy milk (provides 300mg of calcium)
- 175g (6oz) calcium-set tofu (provides 240mg of calcium)
- 150g (5½oz) cooked Asian greens, such as pak choy (provides 125mg of calcium)
- 150g (5½oz) cooked kale (provides 100mg of calcium)
- 150g (5½oz) cooked legumes, such as chickpeas (provides 68mg of calcium)

Iron

Many people rely on red meat for their iron needs, although there are many notable sources of iron from plant foods. Iron is vital for transporting oxygen around the body, energy production, immunity, blood formation and cognitive function.

Animal foods that contain iron

- 65g (2⅛oz) cooked beef, such as lean rump steak (provides 2.2mg of iron)
- 65g (2⅛oz) cooked lamb, such as lean rump steak (provides 2mg of iron)
- 80g (2¾oz) cooked poultry, such as skinless grilled chicken breast (provides 0.6mg of iron)

Plant foods that contain iron

- 170g (6oz) firm tofu (provides 4.9mg of iron)
- 150g (5½oz) legumes, including beans, peas, chickpeas and lentils (provides 2–3mg of iron)
- 100g (3½oz) tempeh (provides 2.7mg of iron)
- 75g (2½oz) cooked spinach (provides 2.7mg of iron)
- 60g (2oz) rolled oats (provides 2.1mg of iron)
- 150g (5½oz) cooked quinoa (provides 1.9mg of iron)
- 30g (2oz) nuts, such as cashews (provides 1.5mg of iron)

The body's absorption of iron from plant foods can be boosted by ensuring iron-rich meals include a good source of vitamin C, such as capsicums, tomatoes or broccoli. Just as iron absorption by the body can be enhanced by vitamin C, it can also be inhibited by phenolic compounds in coffee and black tea, so avoid drinking these with your iron-rich main meals to optimise iron absorption.

Zinc

This mineral performs critical functions in the body, including keeping your immune system fighting fit and maintaining healthy skin, hair and nails. The absorption of zinc is inhibited by phytates, which are compounds found in legumes, wholegrains, nuts and seeds. Not to worry: phytates can be inactivated by food preparation methods including soaking, sprouting (germination) and fermentation, so choosing foods such as wholegrain sourdough bread (which has been fermented) and sprouted seeds will optimise your zinc uptake from meals. The following are good sources of zinc to include in your diet:

Animal foods that contain zinc

- 15g (½oz) fresh oysters (provides 55mg of zinc)
- 65g (2⅛oz) cooked beef, such as lean rump steak (provides 5.3mg of zinc)
- 65g (2⅛oz) cooked lamb, such as lean rump steak (provides 3.8mg of zinc)
- 80g (2¾oz) cooked poultry, such as skinless grilled chicken breast (provides 0.5mg of zinc)

Plant foods that contain zinc

- 170g (6oz) firm tofu (provides 2.9mg of zinc)
- 30g (1oz) seeds, such as pepitas (provides 2.2mg of zinc)
- 30g (1oz) nuts, such as cashews (provides 1.6mg of zinc)
- 150g (5½oz) cooked legumes, including beans, peas, chickpeas and lentils (provides 1–1.5mg of zinc)
- 60g (2oz) rolled oats (provides 1.4mg of zinc)
- 100g (3½oz) tempeh (provides 1.1mg of zinc)

Pumpkin seeds (pepitas) are a good plant food source of zinc, so get into the habit of sprinkling sprouted pumpkin seeds on your meals to boost your zinc intake.

Iodine

The mineral iodine is important for thyroid function, energy metabolism and cognitive function. Most people get a significant proportion of their daily iodine intake from dairy foods, so if you're ditching dairy – particularly cow's milk – it's important to make sure you're getting enough from other sources. Plant foods (with the exception of seaweeds) are a poor source of iodine. A daily multivitamin supplement can be an easy way to ensure you're meeting your iodine needs, which is particularly important if you're planning a pregnancy. Speak to your GP or a dietitian for more information. Here are some good sources of iodine to incorporate into your diet:

Animal foods that contain iodine

- 100g (3½oz) fresh oysters (provides 185mcg of iodine)
- 250ml (9fl oz) cow's milk (provides 60mcg of iodine)
- 2 large eggs (provides 58mcg of iodine)
- 105g (3½oz) canned pink salmon (provides 50mcg of iodine)
- 200g (7oz) natural yogurt (provides 24mcg of iodine)

Plant foods that contain iodine

- ¼ teaspoon (1.5g) iodised salt (provides 66mcg of iodine)
- 2 slices (33g/1¼oz) wheat bread, fortified with iodised salt (provides 33mcg of iodine)

Simple swaps

Going flexitarian involves finding new plant-based favourites to replace the animal products you might have once consumed every day. You may not want to swap out every dairy product in your fridge for a vegan equivalent just yet, but even one or two substitutions will help you towards your personal flexitarian goal. Take a look at this list of healthy plant-based options for common food and drink items to find the right products for you.

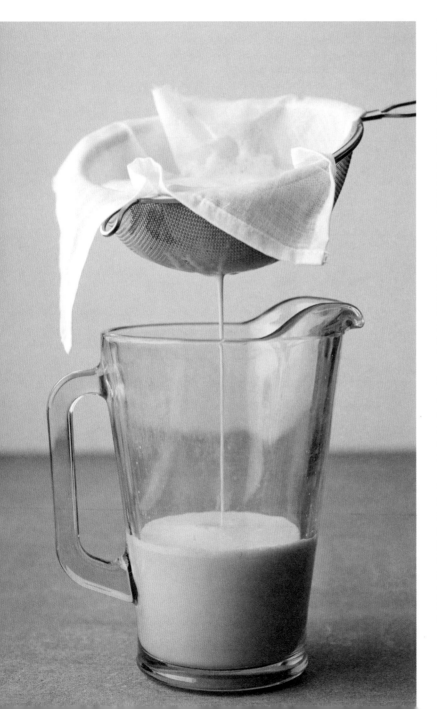

Dairy milk substitutes

Soy milk is made by blending boiled soy beans with water and various additives, such as sugar and calcium. Soy milk has a creamy texture and is great for drinking straight or added to smoothies or cereal. It is also good in tea or coffee as it doesn't split at high temperatures. For this reason, it's also a good choice for cooking and baking. Soy milk is nutritionally the most similar to cow's milk, with around 7 grams of protein per 250ml (9fl oz), but it doesn't contain high amounts of calcium, unless added by the manufacturer, so be sure to check the label.

Unsweetened almond milk is a good alternative to dairy milk in cooking and baking, as well as in smoothies, on cereal, or drinking plain. However, it might add a slight sweetness to savoury dishes (despite the name). Almond milk is produced by blending almonds with water. Not all almond milks are fortified with calcium, so it's important to check the label. Unlike soy milk, almond milk is not a good source of protein.

Unsweetened drinking coconut milk can be drunk on its own, added to cereal, or used in cooking. It is made by combining coconut milk or cream with water, and is found with other long-life milks in supermarkets. It is not nutrient-rich unless fortified by the manufacturer.

Oat milk is made by blending soaked oats and water. It has a slightly viscous texture and mild, sweet taste. It is suitable for drinking plain, in smoothies and in most cooked dishes, except for those that need to be gluten-free. Oat milk is a good source of fibre and also contains the soluble fibre beta-glucan, which is clinically proven to help reduce bad cholesterol levels. It's also a good option for people who have soy or nut allergies.

Rice milk is just rice and water, and has a thin texture due to its low protein content. It's a tasty addition in smoothies or on cereal due to its naturally sweet taste, but it is a significant source of carbohydrates, containing about 30 grams per 250ml (9fl oz). It is another good option for people who have soy or nut allergies.

Butter substitutes

Vegetable oil spreads are ideal for spreading, cooking, or baking. They are a good source of vitamin E, healthy unsaturated fats (including omega-6), and are often fortified with vitamins A and D. It can be used as a substitute for butter weight for weight in recipes. If you are avoiding dairy, be sure to check the label as certain brands contain milk solids.

Cheese substitutes

Nutritional yeast offers a savoury cheese flavour to dishes and is a useful cheese alternative for stirring through risottos and sauces, or for sprinkling over pasta. It is a source of protein and fibre, and is fortified with B vitamins.

Nut cheeses are a blend of nuts and water with a non-dairy probiotic added to ferment the cheese. They are great to use as spreads and to add to cooked dishes, such as lasagne.

You might have noticed the variety of commercial vegan cheeses available in your supermarket. These are usually made with highly processed ingredients, such as soy protein and starches, with the addition of colours and flavours, and are not usually a good source of micronutrients. Of course, you might decide to include these faux cheeses occasionally, but they aren't essential components of a healthy flexitarian diet.

Honey substitutes

Agave nectar is a natural sweetener and has a similar texture to honey. You can swap the honey quantity in a recipe for the same amount of agave.

Rice malt syrup is made from brown rice, giving it a rich flavour with a mild sweetness. It can be substituted for the same amount as honey in recipes.

Maple syrup has a slightly stronger flavour than agave nectar or rice malt syrup. It is great for drizzling and can be substituted for the same amount as honey in recipes. Be sure to purchase pure maple syrup and not an artificial "maple-flavoured" syrup. Maple syrup can be quite expensive, but a little goes a long way.

Meat and seafood substitutes

Tofu is produced by curdling and pressing soy milk. It has a neutral taste and absorbs the flavour of whatever it is marinated or cooked with. Firm tofu is good for using in stir-fries and soups because it keeps its structure, while silken tofu is perfect for making sauces, dressings, and smoothies because it is delicate and falls apart easily. Tofu is a good source of protein, iron, and zinc – and calcium too, if set with the addition of a calcium salt.

Tempeh is a traditional Indonesian food that is made by fermenting soy beans into a savoury cake form. It has a strong nutty flavour and a chewy texture, making it a great addition to stir-fries. It is even higher in protein than tofu, and is a good source of iron and zinc.

Seitan is a non-soy product, made from vital wheat gluten and water to form a dough which is usually shaped to resemble meat or seafood and then cooked. It has a meaty and chewy texture with a similar "bite" to chicken, and can be used as a substitute for meat or fish in cooked dishes. Seitan is a good source of protein, iron, and zinc.

As well as a plethora of commercial vegan cheeses that are now available in supermarkets, you'll also notice a variety of faux meat and seafood products. These are usually highly processed and full of artificial ingredients and aren't essential to a healthy flexitarian diet.

Egg substitutes

Aquafaba is the liquid that chickpeas have been cooked in, and includes the liquid from a can of chickpeas. It has emulsifying, binding, foaming, and thickening properties and is the perfect substitute for egg whites in recipes that call for beaten egg whites, such as meringues and chocolate mousse. In general, three tablespoons of aquafaba is equal to one egg.

Chia seeds mixed with water are a good swap for eggs in baking recipes, as the mixture works like a binding agent similar to eggs. A mixture of one tablespoon of chia seeds to three tablespoons of water is equal to one egg.

Flax seeds and water can be used in the same way as chia seeds to replace egg, but this mixture has a stronger and nuttier flavour.

The flexitarian storecupboard

The secret to any diet change is not to be caught short, or else you can quickly revert to old ways. Flexitarianism is no different. Make sure to keep your storecupboard well-stocked with items such as those listed here, focusing on nutritious wholefoods in their natural, unprocessed state wherever possible.

Baking ingredients

Baking powder and bicarbonate of soda for making cakes, biscuits, brownies, and muffins.

Cocoa or raw cacao powder to use in baked goods, smoothies, or hot chocolate.

Flours such as wholemeal, plain, and self-raising flours, plus gluten-free varieties (such as buckwheat) if required.

Good-quality dark chocolate (either in block form or as chips) to use in baking. If you're limiting your dairy intake, be sure to choose a vegan variety.

Sweeteners, including maple syrup, agave nectar, rice malt syrup, and raw brown sugar.

Savoury staples

A selection of dried herbs and spices are essential for everyday cooking. Useful ones to have on hand include bay leaves, pepper, cayenne pepper, cinnamon, coriander, cumin, curry powder, chilli, ginger, mustard seeds, nutmeg, oregano, smoked paprika, salt, thyme, turmericn and rosemary.

Canned black beans and kidney beans are a good meat alternative for homemade burgers, stews and Mexican-inspired dishes.

Canned cannellini beans are perfect in soups, salads or simply mashed with garlic, lemon, and herbs to use as a spread or dip.

Canned chickpeas are an essential storecupboard item in a flexitarian diet. Affordable and a great source of protein, they can be used to whip up a quick hummus dip, to make falafels or as an addition to salads, pasta dishes and curries.

Canned lentils are a nutritious replacement for minced meat in Italian recipes, such as spaghetti Bolognese, and are perfect for salads, soups, and curries.

Dried versions of the above legumes are cheaper than canned for when you have time to soak them prior to cooking.

Green and yellow split peas to add a smoky flavour to soups and dhals.

Other legumes, such as mung beans, borlotti beans, adzuki beans, black beans, moth beans, haricot beans, pigeon peas, black-eyed beans, pinto beans and soy beans, can be purchased as required and as you grow more confident in trying out new foods and recipes.

Nuts, seeds, and dried fruits

Almonds and cashews are storecupboard essentials, as they are perfect for baking, making "cheese" fillings and nut milks and for plain old snacking.

Chia seeds and flaxseeds can be added to porridge, cereal, muesli, and smoothies. Mixed with water, they act as an ideal egg replacment when baking.

Dried fruits, such as Medjool dates, raisins, figs and apricots, come in handy when making muesli or baking, and they make marvellous snacks, too.

Pumpkin, sesame, and sunflower seeds are good garnishes to keep on hand to add a crunch to salads, soups, and stir-fries.

Walnuts, pecans, and pine nuts are delicious, especially when toasted first, and great to have on hand for snacking and baking.

Oils

Extra-virgin olive oil (preferably cold-pressed) is perfect for drizzling over Mediterranean dishes and whisked into salad dressings. Extra-virgin olive oil has a relatively high smoke point, so should not be used for frying.

Olive oil is better suited to quick frying and roasting than extra-virgin olive oil (see above).

Rapeseed oil is light and clear with a neutral flavour; it is a good choice for quick frying.

Coconut oil is great in curries and baked goods, but use in moderation as it is high in saturated fat.

Sesame oil adds a nutty flavour to Asian dishes, and is an excellent addition to marinades and sauces.

Sunflower and vegetable oils have a high smoke point and are best used for deep-frying dishes.

Grain-based foods

Grains such as brown rice, quinoa, bulgur, freekah, wholegrain couscous, and pearl barley.

Rolled oats to make porridge, muesli, granola, and baked goods.

Wholegrain sourdough bread to top with healthy spreads or make sandwiches.

Wholemeal dried pasta and ramen, soba, and rice noodles for easy weeknight dinners.

Staples and condiments

Canned staples such as whole and diced tomatoes, coconut milk, and coconut cream.

Dried staples such as nutritional yeast and breadcrumbs.

Olives, pickled cucumbers, capers, sundried tomatoes, or preserved artichoke hearts to add flavour to meals.

Sauces and pastes, including a good-quality homemade or shop-bought tomato sauce, a hot chilli sauce such as sriracha or sambal oelek, good-quality curry pastes, tomato paste, harissa paste, Worcestershire sauce, fish sauce (vegan varieties are available), hoisin sauce, salsa, soy sauce, kecap manis (sweet soy sauce), and tamari (Japanese soy sauce).

Spreads such as peanut butter, almond butter, tahini, Marmite, jams, marmalades, and mustard.

Soy milk or your other favourite plant-based non-dairy milk, such as coconut, almond, or oat.

Vinegars for dressings and sauces, such as balsamic, apple cider, rice wine, and red wine vinegars.

Frozen foods

Frozen berries are just as nutritious as fresh berries but with the convenience of staying fresher for longer. Ensure you buy a brand that doesn't add sugar – check the ingredients list on the packet if you are unsure.

Frozen vegetables, such as peas, sweetcorn, and spinach, are handy for soups and stews.

Meal planning

A flexitarian diet is, of course, designed to be flexible. Nevertheless, getting into the habit of meal planning will make meeting your goals a lot easier. Put aside a little time each week to decide what you're going to cook (and whether they'll include meat or fish) and you'll save time and effort in the long run.

Below is a sample weekly menu made up of recipes from this book. Decide in advance which recipes will include animal products, write up a shopping list for all the ingredients you'll need, and remember to include a nutritious snack or two every day (such as a handful of nuts or a piece of fresh fruit), and your week will be full of delicious healthy food.

Freeze any leftovers and you'll soon have a freezer stocked with meals for busy weeks when your cooking time is limited.

	Breakfast	Lunch	Dinner
Monday	Wheat Grain Bircher Muesli Pots (page 64) can be made in advance and will keep in the fridge for quick breakfasts or snacks throughout the week.	Savoury Green Pancakes with Feta and Sprout Salad (page 88). These can be made over the weekend so they are ready for weekday lunches.	Rainbow Lentil Meatballs with Arrabbiata Sauce (page 220)
Tuesday	Spiced Apple and Mung Bean Muffins (page 58) are perfect for breakfast or snacks throughout the week.	Quinoa Falafel with Mint Yogurt Sauce (page 106)	Black-eyed Bean Sliders with Pico de Gallo (page 94)
Wednesday	Wheat Grain Bircher Muesli Pots (page 64)	Mung Bean Gado Gado (page 120)	Butter Bean Enchiladas (page 204)
Thursday	Curried Mung Bean Avocado Toast (page 46)	Rainbow Bowl with Sesame and Ginger Dressing (page 114)	Green Minestrone with Kale and Walnut Pesto (page 152), making a double batch for lunch tomorrow.
Friday	Tropical Smoothie Bowl (page 60)	Green Minestrone with Kale and Walnut Pesto (page 152), using leftovers from last night's dinner.	Courgette, Herb and Lemon Tagine (page 184)
Saturday	Black Bean Breakfast Tostadas (page 54)	Avocado, Coriander and Lime Tabbouleh (page 124)	Brazilian Black Bean and Pumpkin Stew (page 160), making a double batch for lunch tomorrow.
Sunday	Wholemeal Pancakes with Apple and Cinnamon (page 62)	Brazilian Black Bean and Pumpkin Stew (page 160), using leftovers from last night's dinner.	Shaved Asparagus, Mint and Edamame Spaghetti (page 212)

Basics

There's nothing quite like using your own homemade basics when cooking. Make your own stock, nut milk, yogurt, fresh pasta dough and more with these essential recipes.

Simple Vegetable Stock

This light and flavourful vegetable stock blends well with all manner of other ingredients, making it the perfect base for any soup or sauce.

makes 4 litres (7 pints) **prep** 15 mins **cook** 2 hours

1 In a large stockpot or deep-sided large pan, combine the leeks, onions, carrots, celery, button mushrooms, bay leaf, flat-leaf parsley, thyme, peppercorns and tamari. Cover with the filtered water.

2 Set the pan over a high heat, bring to the boil, cover, reduce the heat to a gentle simmer and cook for 2 hours.

3 Cool completely; strain and discard the vegetables, herbs and spices; and pour the stock into glass jars or BPA-free containers for storage. Stock will keep in the fridge for up to 7 days or in the freezer for up to 3 months.

2 large leeks, halved lengthways, washed, and cut into 2.5cm (1in) chunks

2 large brown onions, root end trimmed and cut into 2.5cm (1in) chunks

4 carrots, scrubbed and cut into 2.5cm (1in) chunks

8 large sticks celery, cut into 2.5cm (1in) chunks

140g (5oz) button mushrooms, sliced

1 bay leaf

30g (1oz) fresh flat-leaf parsley leaves and stems

3 sprigs thyme

1 tsp whole black peppercorns

2 tbsp tamari or soy sauce

4 litres (7 pints) filtered water

Why not try...

For Mushroom Stock, sauté the leeks, carrots and celery in 2 tbsp extra-virgin olive oil for 15 minutes or until golden. Add 140g (5oz) sliced chestnut mushrooms and 25g (scant 1oz) dried porcini mushrooms to the pan along with raw, unpeeled onions when you add water, and proceed as directed.

Vegan Ramen Stock

This stock is light and fragrant, and will provide the perfect base for ramen. Charring the onion and ginger will increase their flavour profiles. Do it over an open flame or in a dry pan over a high heat.

makes 1.4–1.7 litres (2½–2¾ pints) **prep** 15 mins **cook** 45 mins

1 Heat the vegetable oil in a large pot over a medium-high heat. Add the onion, celery, ginger, leeks, carrots, and garlic.

2 Stirring constantly, cook for 10 minutes to caramelize the vegetables.

3 Add the water and bring to the boil over a high heat. Add the button mushrooms and spring onions, lower the heat to a simmer, and cook for 30 minutes.

4 Allow to cool to room temperature, or overnight in the fridge to allow maximum infused flavour. Strain the stock and discard the solids. Stock will keep in the fridge for up to 7 days or in the freezer for up to 3 months.

2 tbsp vegetable oil

1 large onion, roughly chopped

2 celery stalks, roughly chopped

5cm (2in) knob ginger, sliced

2 leeks, sliced and washed

2 large carrots, roughly chopped (no need to peel)

6–8 medium cloves of garlic, crushed

2 litres (3½ pints) water

175g (6oz) button mushrooms, roughly chopped

1 bunch spring onions (6–8 stems), roughly chopped

Fresh Pasta Dough

You can easily make your own fresh pasta dough with or without eggs. For added flavour and a pretty golden colour, try saffron or tomato paste – or both. Use a pasta machine to roll the dough if you have one, but a rolling pin also works well if you don't.

serves 4   **prep** 30 mins   **cook** 3 mins

1 In a small bowl, whisk the extra-virgin olive oil into the warm water. Then, whisk in the tomato puree and/or saffron (if using).

2 In a large bowl, stir together the flour and salt. Mound the flour mixture on a wooden board or clean kitchen worktop, and make a well in the centre. Pour the olive oil–water mixture into the well.

3 Using a fork, slowly whisk the flour mixture into the olive oil mixture, a little at a time, until nearly all has been incorporated. Knead by hand for about 5 minutes, sprinkling your work surface with flour as you work. If the dough seems dry, add more water, a few drops at a time. When you've finished kneading, you should end up with a pliable ball of dough that's firm, yet springy when pressed.

4 Wrap the ball of dough in cling wrap, and rest at room temperature for 20 minutes. Meanwhile, prepare the pasta machine or dust a rolling pin and work surface with flour.

5 Using your fingers, press the dough into a rectangle. Follow the instructions that came with your pasta machine, rolling the dough until it's thin but no longer opaque. Or use a rolling pin to roll the dough into a large rectangle, turning it a quarter-turn clockwise with each roll and flipping it over several times. Dust the board with flour frequently to prevent sticking.

6 Cut the pasta sheets into your desired shape, or fill, and cook in boiling, well-salted water for about 3 minutes or until tender. Serve immediately with your favourite sauce.

2 tbsp extra-virgin olive oil

240ml (8fl oz) warm water

1 tsp tomato puree and/or a pinch of saffron crushed in a mortar and pestle (optional)

450g (1lb) plain flour, plus more for kneading

½ tsp sea salt

Make it vegetarian

Replace 240ml (8fl oz) warm water with 4 eggs. Mix the eggs with the olive oil in Step 1 and pour the mixture into the well in Step 2.

Pie Pastry

This easy pastry comes together quickly in the food processor. It yields a flaky, tender pie crust and works equally well for both sweet and savoury recipes.

makes 2 crusts for a deep-dish pie   **prep** 10 mins, plus 30 mins chilling time   **cook** none

1 In a food processor fitted with a metal blade, pulse the flour and salt several times to combine.

2 Add half of the vegetable oil spread cubes, pulse 5 or 6 times, and process for 5 seconds. Add remaining vegetable oil spread and pulse until the mixture forms small, pea-sized pieces.

3 Transfer the flour mixture to a large bowl. Pour a few tablespoons of iced water over the flour mix, and quickly toss with a large kitchen fork to combine. Continue adding the water and tossing until the mixture just comes together and then use the heel of your hand to press the dough against the sides of the bowl to form a moist, cohesive ball.

4 Separate the dough into two equal pieces, wrap in cling film and use your hands to flatten each piece into a 12cm (5in) disc.

5 Chill the dough for 30 minutes and proceed as directed in your recipe.

375g (13oz) unbleached plain flour

1½ tsp sea salt

12 tbsp vegetable oil spread, partially frozen, cut into small cubes (or solid coconut oil)

120–150ml (4–5fl oz) iced water

Make it vegetarian

Instead of vegetable oil spread or coconut oil, simply use dairy butter.

Nut Milk

Once you've tasted homemade nut milk, you'll never go back to shop-bought.

serves 4 **prep** 5 mins, plus overnight soaking time **cook** none

1 Soak almonds in cold water overnight.

2 Discard the soaking water, rinse the nuts well and drain.

3 In a high-speed blender, process the nuts along with the filtered water, Medjool dates, vanilla extract and cinnamon until smooth.

4 Using a nut milk bag or muslin bag, strain the solids from the milk into a clean glass jar.

5 Refrigerate the milk for up to 4 days. Shake well before using.

140g (5oz) raw almonds, hazelnuts or cashews

960ml (1¾ pints) filtered water

2 or 3 pitted Medjool dates

1 tsp vanilla extract

½ tsp ground cinnamon

Why not try...

For Chocolate Nut Milk, add 25g (scant 1oz) raw cacao and 1 tbsp agave nectar to the blender with the other ingredients.

Nut Butter

When properly soaked, dried nuts are easy to turn into delicious nut butter. Far better than anything from the supermarket, this nut butter is packed with healthy fat, protein and energy.

makes about 30 servings of 2 tbsp   **prep** 10 minutes, plus overnight soaking time   **cook** none

1   Soak nuts in cold water overnight.

2   Discard the soaking water, rinse the nuts well and drain. In a food processor fitted with a metal chopping blade, pulse the nuts until they resemble flour.

3   Add the coconut oil and sea salt, and process, stopping to scrape down the sides of the bowl as needed, until the nut butter has reached your desired consistency.

4   Transfer the nut butter to a glass jar, seal tightly, and store in the fridge for up to 6 months.

500g (1lb 2oz) raw nuts

4 tbsp coconut oil, melted

⅛ tsp sea salt

Nut Cheese

If you're cutting back on dairy, nut cheese – which can be spreadable or hard in texture – is a tasty substitute.

makes about 250g (9oz)   **prep** 15 minutes, plus overnight soaking time   **cook** none

1   Soak nuts in cold water with 1 tsp of sea salt overnight.

2   Discard the soaking water, rinse the nuts well and drain. In a high-speed blender, process the nuts, coconut oil, lemon juice, garlic and ⅛ tsp of sea salt for 5-7 minutes, or until smooth.

3   Transfer the mixture to a nut milk bag, or a colander lined with cheesecloth, press down on the solids or squeeze to remove the excess liquid, and form the cheese into a ball.

4   Serve immediately, for a creamier cheese. For a harder cheese, chill in the fridge for 24 hours before serving.

150g (5½oz) raw cashews or almonds

1⅛ tsp sea salt

180ml (6fl oz) water

2 tbsp coconut oil, melted

3 tsp lemon juice

1 garlic clove

Yogurt

Tangy, silky yogurt is easy to make and much healthier than shop-bought versions. Add soaked and dried nuts or unsweetened, flaked coconut, and season with cinnamon and nutmeg for a nutritious snack.

serves 8   **prep** 2 mins   **cook** 24 hours

1 In a medium saucepan over a low heat, heat the milk for about 10 minutes, or until it reaches 80°C (175°F). Use a thermometer. If you're using raw milk, heat it to 40°C (100°F).

2 Remove from the heat, and allow the milk to cool for about 10 minutes, or until it reaches 40°C (100°F).

3 Place the commercial yogurt in a 1-litre (1¾ pint) glass jar with a tight-fitting lid, and fill the jar with warm milk, leaving 2.5cm (1in) space at the top.

4 Place the jar in a yogurt maker or a dehydrator set to 40°C (100°F), or in the oven with the light on for 24 hours.

5 Allow the yogurt to cool in the fridge.

950ml (1¾ pints) organic, raw or lightly pasteurised unhomogenised whole milk

60ml (2fl oz) organic commercial yogurt

Make it vegan

Substitute one 400ml (14fl oz) can of coconut milk for the organic whole milk. Shake the can vigorously before opening. Add 1 probiotic capsule to the coconut milk, and culture as directed.

Vegan Mayonnaise

You can easily find vegan mayonnaise at the supermarket, but this simple recipe will have you making your own in no time! The soy milk helps with thickening, allowing you to replicate the smooth texture of mayonnaise.

makes 250ml (9fl oz) **prep** 5 mins **cook** none

1 Combine all the ingredients except the oil in a high-speed blender and blend on high for 1 minute.

2 Reduce the speed to low and slowly pour in the oil until the mixture begins to thicken.

3 Taste the mayonnaise and adjust accordingly. Add more oil for a creamier mayonnaise, or add more mustard, agave nectar, vinegar or salt to taste.

120ml (4fl oz) unsweetened soy milk

1 tsp apple cider vinegar

juice of ½ lemon (1 tbsp)

½ tsp agave nectar (or sweetener of your choice)

½ tsp Dijon mustard

¾ tsp salt

250ml (9fl oz) grapeseed oil (or any neutral-tasting vegetable oil)

Why not try...

You can also try using silken tofu to make vegan mayonnaise. Replace the soy milk in this recipe with 225g (8oz) silken tofu and use only 3 tbsp grapeseed oil. Drain the tofu and transfer to a blender. Add the remaining ingredients and blend until smooth and creamy.

Tofu

While widely considered a health food, tofu is a staple of both vegetarian and Japanese diets. You can find tofu in many different varieties: silken, soft, firm and extra firm. Tofu is made from mature soy beans that have been dried (known as daizu), as well as nigari, which acts as a coagulant (solidifier). If you'd like fresh firm tofu to add to your flexitarian meals, simply follow these steps.

makes 400g (14oz) **prep** 1 hour, plus overnight soaking time **cook** 20 mins

1 In a large bowl filled with 1 litre of water, soak the dried soy beans overnight, about 8–12 hours.

2 In a food processor, grind the soy beans and soaking water for 2 minutes, or until fine.

3 In a large pan over a medium heat, bring 1.2 litres (2 pints) of water to the boil. Add the ground soy beans and stir continuously with a wooden spatula. Just before the mixture comes to the boil, reduce the heat to low and cook, stirring continuously, for 8 minutes.

4 Line a colander with finely woven cotton cloth, and place over a large pan. Strain the mixture through the cloth, and discard the solids.

5 Cook the soy milk strained into the pan over a low heat, stirring continuously with the wooden spatula. When the temperature registers between 66–68°C (151–154°F), remove the pan from the heat.

6 In a small bowl filled with 6 tablespoons of lukewarm water, dissolve the nigari.

7 Add half of the nigari mixture to the soy milk, stirring with the spatula in a whirlpool pattern. While the soy milk is swirling, add the remaining nigari mixture, stirring gently afterwards in a figure-of-eight pattern. You should notice the soy milk beginning to coagulate. Cover the pan, and leave to stand for 15 minutes.

8 Line a colander with a tightly woven cotton cloth (don't reuse the previous one), and set over a bowl that can support it. With a soup ladle, gently transfer the coagulated soy milk to the cloth-lined colander.

9 Fold the cloth over top of the coagulated soy milk, and place a weight on top. Leave to stand for 15 minutes.

10 Remove the weight and gently transfer the bowl to a sink filled with cold water to cool. Once chilled, unfold the cloth, and gently lift out the finished tofu.

11 Use the tofu immediately, or store in an airtight container with fresh, cold water in the fridge for up to 1 week.

200g (7oz) dried soy beans

2 tsp nigari (found in Japanese supermarkets or health food stores)

Béchamel Sauce

Smooth béchamel is the perfect choice when a creamy sauce is desired. A hint of onion, clove and nutmeg adds just a bit of spice to this delicious and versatile sauce.

makes 480ml (16fl oz)   **prep** 5 mins   **cook** 10-15 mins

1   Heat the grapeseed oil in a small saucepan over a medium–high heat. Add the flour all at once and stir vigorously with a whisk.

2   When the flour mixture is golden and begins to smell nutty (but before it browns, about 2 minutes), add the non-dairy milk, continuing to whisk vigorously to prevent lumps.

3   Add the clove-studded onion and bay leaf, reduce the heat to low, and cook, stirring frequently, for about 10 minutes or until the sauce thickens.

4   Remove from the heat, and stir in salt, black pepper and nutmeg. Taste and adjust seasonings.

5   Strain the sauce through a fine-mesh sieve to remove any solids, and use immediately.

4 tbsp grapeseed oil

3 tbsp plain flour

600ml (1 pint) unflavoured non-dairy milk, preferably soy or rice

¼ small onion, studded with 1 whole clove

1 bay leaf

¼ tsp sea salt

pinch freshly ground black pepper

pinch freshly grated nutmeg

Make it vegetarian

If you'd like a dairy béchamel sauce, replace the grapeseed oil with butter and the non-dairy milk with cow's milk.

Mushroom Gravy

This rich, brown, flavourful gravy never disappoints. Using a deep, wondrous mushroom stock (see page 30) and taking time to cook the roux without burning it are the secrets to this great gravy.

makes 960ml (1¾ pints) **prep** 10 mins **cook** 30 mins

1 Heat 3 tablespoons of the grapeseed oil in a medium frying pan over a medium–high heat, until it shimmers (but before it begins to smoke). Add the shallots and cook, stirring occasionally, for about 5 minutes or until softened.

2 Add the garlic, both lots of mushrooms, and cook, stirring often, for 10 minutes or until the mushrooms have released their liquid.

3 Add the mushroom stock and tamari, reduce the heat to medium, and cook, stirring occasionally, while you make the roux.

4 In a small pan over a medium heat, heat the remaining 2 tablespoons of grapeseed oil. Whisk in the flour and cook, stirring frequently, for about 10 minutes or until the mixture is a rich brown colour.

5 Whisk the roux into the mushroom mixture, and cook for a further 5-10 minutes or until the gravy is as thick as you like it. Stir in bourbon (if using) and black pepper, and serve immediately. This gravy will keep in a tightly sealed container in the fridge for 3 days.

5 tbsp grapeseed oil

2 medium shallots, finely chopped

1 clove garlic, smashed and finely chopped

225g (8oz) chestnut mushrooms, thinly sliced

225g (8oz) shiitake mushrooms, thinly sliced

960ml (1¾ pints) Mushroom Stock (see page 30)

1 tbsp salt-reduced tamari or soy sauce

3 tbsp plain flour

1 tbsp bourbon (optional)

½ tsp freshly ground black pepper

Tomato Sauce

This simple, fresh-tasting tomato sauce comes together in minutes. Use the best-quality canned tomatoes you can find for this quick and easy sauce that's perfect with pasta or as a base for soup.

makes 840ml (1½ pints) **prep** 5 mins **cook** 15 mins

1 Heat the olive oil in a large saucepan over a medium–high heat. When the oil is shimmering (but before it begins to smoke), add the garlic and salt. Cook, stirring, for 30 seconds, to allow the garlic to release its fragrance without browning.

2 Add the tomatoes with their juice and the white wine to the pan, and cook for 5 minutes.

3 Using a potato masher or a large fork, crush the tomatoes. Reduce the heat to medium and cook, stirring occasionally, for a further 10 minutes.

4 Stir in the basil and black pepper, and remove from the heat.

5 Use immediately, or pour into freezer-safe containers with 2.5cm (1in) headspace and freeze for up to 3 months.

2 tbsp extra-virgin olive oil

2 cloves garlic, peeled, smashed and finely chopped

½ tsp sea salt

2 (400g) cans peeled tomatoes, with juice

4 tbsp dry white wine

4 leaves fresh basil, torn

¼ tsp freshly ground black pepper

Breakfasts

Break up your usual breakfast routine with these delicious, modern recipes. Some are perfect for leisurely brunches, while others can be made ahead for a no-fuss midweek breakfast.

Curried Mung Bean Avocado Toast

Sprouts and mung beans elevate avocado toast to the next level of tasty. The hint of curry flavour adds extra depth to the creamy, smooth avocado.

makes 3   **prep** 10 mins   **cook** 4 mins

1 In a frying pan over a medium-low heat, toast the bread for 2 minutes on each side, or until brown and crisp. Remove from the frying pan and let cool slightly.

2 Cut the avocado in half and remove the pit. Scoop the flesh from one half and add to a medium mixing bowl. Mash the avocado half with a potato masher.

3 Stir in the mung beans, curry powder, and turmeric. Season with salt and pepper to taste. Spread the avocado mixture evenly over the slices of toast.

4 Remove the flesh from the remaining avocado half and slice thinly. Arrange equal amounts on each slice of toast.

5 Place on serving plates and sprinkle with the beansprouts and chives. Serve immediately.

3 slices of sourdough or wholewheat bread

1 ripe avocado

175g (6oz) cooked mung beans

½ tsp curry powder

pinch of turmeric

salt and freshly ground black pepper

45g (1½oz) sprouted mung beans (beansprouts)

3 tbsp chopped chives

Make it with meat

Crumble 2 rashers of cooked crispy bacon into the avocado–mung bean mixture.

Lentil Cream Cheese Tartines

Flavoured cream cheese is very easy to make at home. Adding lentils, chives and lemon zest provides texture and some extra protein to this simple breakfast dish.

makes 6   **prep** 5 mins   **cook** 25 mins

1   Preheat the oven to 150°C (300°F). Arrange the slices of bread on a baking sheet. Toast for 5 minutes, turn over, and toast for another 5 minutes until crisp and golden.

2   Meanwhile, to make the cream cheese spread, in a food processor blend the cream cheese, lentils, chives, and lemon zest until thoroughly combined. Season with salt and pepper to taste. Spread the mixture evenly over the slices of toast.

3   In a non-stick frying pan, heat 1 teaspoon of oil over a medium-low heat until shimmering. Crack 2 eggs into the frying pan and cook for 2–3 minutes until the whites are set but the yolks are runny. Place each egg atop a slice of toast then repeat with the remaining 4 eggs. Top each tartine with watercress and serve immediately.

6 slices wholewheat bread

225g (8oz) cream cheese, softened

100g (3½oz) cooked brown lentils

2 tbsp chopped chives

zest of 1 lemon

salt and freshly ground black pepper

3 tsp olive oil

6 large eggs

115g (4oz) watercress

Make it vegan

Use a nut cheese (see page 37) instead of cream cheese and omit the eggs from this recipe.

Make it with fish

Top each tartine with 30g (1oz) thinly sliced smoked salmon.

Roasted Tomato and Chickpea Frittata

Frittatas are a wonderful way to feed a crowd for breakfast or brunch. Chickpeas add an unexpected twist and extra body to this morning classic.

serves 10   **prep** 15 mins   **cook** 30 mins

1   Preheat the oven to 200°C (400°F). On a baking tray, toss the tomatoes, garlic, and thyme in the oil. Spread in an even layer and roast for 10 minutes. Discard the thyme. Let cool slightly.

2   Meanwhile, in a large mixing bowl whisk together the eggs, double cream, and chives. Season with salt and pepper.

3   Heat a 25cm (10in) cast-iron or ovenproof frying pan over a medium heat. Transfer the tomatoes to the frying pan. Add the spinach and cook for 1–2 minutes until the spinach slightly wilts. Add the chickpeas and stir to combine. Spread the mixture evenly across the frying pan.

4   Pour the egg mixture over the tomatoes, spinach, and chickpeas. Cook uncovered for 2–3 minutes, until the edges of the egg begin to set. Transfer the frying pan to the oven and cook uncovered for an additional 8–10 minutes, until the edges are firm but the centre is still slightly springy. Serve immediately.

450g (1lb) baby plum tomatoes

1 garlic clove, finely chopped

2 sprigs of thyme

1 tbsp olive oil

10 large eggs

2 tbsp double cream

2 tsp chopped chives

salt and freshly ground black pepper

85g (3oz) baby spinach

350g (12oz) cooked chickpeas

Why not try...

For a creamy tang, sprinkle 115g (4oz) goat's cheese over the egg mixture before baking.

Make it with meat

Add 140g (5oz) finely diced cooked ham or chicken sausage to the frying pan with the chickpeas in step 3.

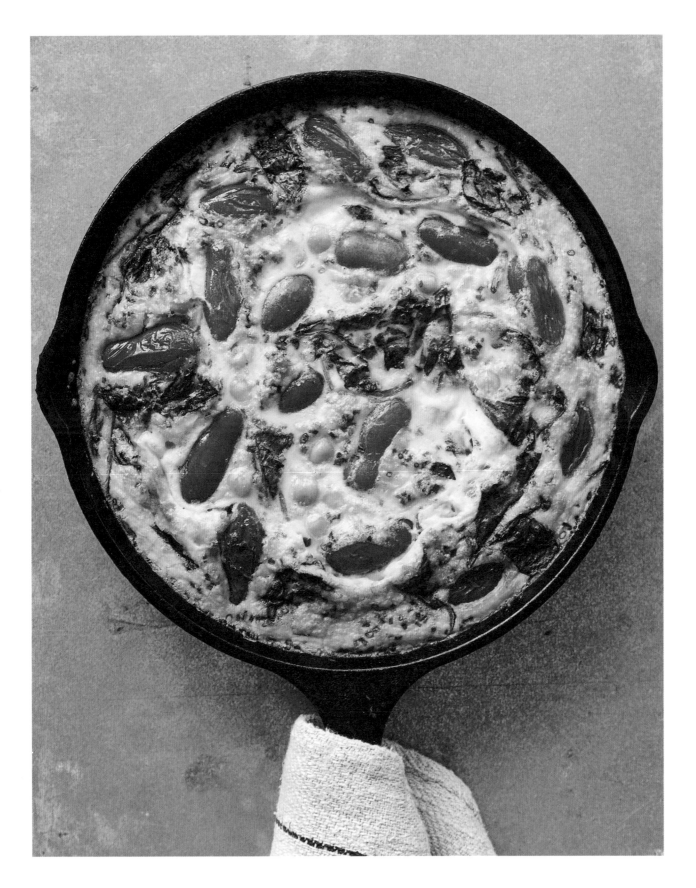

Spinach and Artichoke Quiche

This tasty quiche uses amaranth flour for a delicious crust and is ideal for a healthy and filling brunch. For best results, use artichokes that have been preserved in oil instead of those canned in water or brine.

serves 6   **prep** 20 mins   **cook** 50 mins

1   Preheat the oven to 200°C (400°F/Gas 6). Grease a 22cm (9in) loose-bottomed flan tin and set aside. For the pastry, place both lots of flour, almonds, and salt in a large bowl and mix well until combined. In a small bowl, whisk together the oil and 3 tablespoons of water. Make a well in the centre of the dry ingredients and pour the oil mixture in. Bring together to form a light and sticky dough, adding more water, a little at a time, if needed.

2   Roll out the dough between two sheets of cling film and use to line the prepared tin, making sure it forms a good side to the case. Prick the bottom of the pastry with a fork. Place in the oven and blind bake for about 10 minutes. Then remove from the heat and set aside. Reduce the oven temperature to 180°C (350°F/Gas 4).

3   For the filling, heat the oil in a large saucepan over a medium heat. Add the garlic and onions and cook for about 3-5 minutes or until the onions are translucent. Then add the spinach and cook for a further 2-3 minutes or until it has wilted. Remove from the heat and set aside.

4   For the custard, place the eggs, yolks, and milk in a large bowl. Season with ¼ teaspoon salt and a good grinding of pepper. Whisk until well combined. Spoon the onion and spinach mixture into the pastry case, making sure it covers the bottom. Spread out the artichoke hearts on top in a single layer and pour over the custard. Crumble the cheese and sprinkle over the custard.

5   Bake the quiche in the oven for about 40 minutes or until the custard has set and the top is golden. Remove from the heat and leave to cool slightly before cutting into wedges to serve. This quiche can be served warm or at room temperature.

For the pastry

70g (2¼oz) amaranth flour

45g (1½oz) tapioca flour or cornflour

30g (1oz) ground almonds

¼ tsp salt

3 tbsp sunflower oil

For the filling

1 tbsp olive oil

1 garlic clove, crushed

110g (3¾oz) onion, finely chopped

140g (5oz) spinach

4-5 artichoke hearts, drained and roughly chopped

60g (2oz) goat's cheese

For the custard

2 large eggs

2 egg yolks

250ml (9fl oz) whole milk

salt and freshly ground black pepper

Black Bean Breakfast Tostadas

These crunchy fried tortillas are topped with creamy scrambled eggs and spicy, savoury black beans for an irresistible Mexican-style breakfast.

serves 4　**prep** 15 mins　**cook** 20 mins

1 Preheat the oven to 170°C (325°F). In a medium frying pan, heat the oil over a medium-low heat. Add the onion and cook for 5 minutes, or until translucent. Add the jalapeño and garlic and cook for an additional 2–3 minutes.

2 Add the black beans, cumin, and chipotle chilli powder and stir to coat. Add the stock, bring to the boil, then reduce to a simmer and cook for 5 minutes, or until the liquid reduces. Season with salt and pepper to taste.

3 Meanwhile, arrange the tostada shells on a baking tray in an even layer, with their edges slightly overlapping. Bake for 2–3 minutes until warmed through.

4 In a small mixing bowl, whisk together the eggs and double cream. In a non-stick frying pan, over a medium-low heat, scramble the eggs to the desired consistency.

5 To assemble, spread equal amounts of the black bean mixture on the tostada shells. Top with equal amounts of scrambled eggs. Sprinkle a quarter of the feta on each tostada, then garnish with coriander and hot sauce. Serve immediately.

1 tbsp olive oil

1 small onion, finely diced

1 jalapeño, deseeded and finely diced

1 garlic clove, finely chopped

350g (12oz) cooked black beans

1 tbsp ground cumin

1 tsp chipotle chilli powder

120ml (4fl oz) vegetable stock

salt and freshly ground black pepper

4 corn tostada shells

4 large eggs

½ tbsp double cream

115g (4oz) feta cheese

sprigs of coriander, to garnish

hot sauce, to garnish

Why not try...

For a boost of healthy fats, top each tostada with wedges of sliced avocado.

Make it vegan

Instead of eggs and double cream, scramble 225g (8oz) firm tofu with salt and pepper. For the feta, use a nut cheese (see page 37).

Make it with meat

Crumble 1 rasher of crispy bacon over the beans as you assemble the tostadas.

Asparagus and Green Lentils with Poached Egg

This impressive-looking brunch dish couldn't be easier to prepare. The yolk from the poached egg makes a luxurious sauce for the roasted asparagus and lentils.

serves 4   **prep** 10 mins   **cook** 15 mins

1   Preheat the oven to 180°C (350°F). Toss the asparagus with 1 tablespoon of oil. Arrange on a baking tray in a single layer and season with salt and pepper. Roast for 10 minutes, or until tender.

2   Meanwhile, to make the dressing, in a medium bowl combine the red wine vinegar, Dijon mustard, thyme, and remaining 1 tablespoon of oil. Whisk until emulsified. Add the lentils and stir to combine. Set aside and let the lentils absorb the dressing.

3   To poach the eggs, fill a large saucepan with water, about 4cm (1½in) deep. Bring to the boil then reduce to a simmer. Add the white vinegar. One at a time, crack each egg into a ramekin and gently tip it into the water. Cook for 3 minutes. Drain and place on a plate lined with kitchen paper.

4   To serve, divide the asparagus among 4 plates and top each with the lentils. Place 1 poached egg atop the lentils. Season with pepper and serve immediately.

450g (1lb) fine asparagus, woody ends trimmed

2 tbsp olive oil

salt and freshly ground black pepper

2½ tbsp red wine vinegar

1 tbsp Dijon mustard

¼ tsp chopped thyme

⅛ tsp of white vinegar

400g (14oz) cooked green lentils

4 large eggs

Make it with meat

Add 1 slice of Parma ham or a rasher of crispy bacon to each plate.

Spiced Apple and Mung Bean Muffins

Mung beans pureed with apple sauce make for one of the moistest muffins you'll ever taste and provide protein and fibre for a filling on-the-go breakfast.

serves 12 **prep** 35 mins **cook** 20 mins

1 Preheat the oven to 175°C (350°F). In a food processor, combine the apple sauce, mung beans, and agave. Purée until smooth.

2 In a large mixing bowl, whisk together the wholemeal flour, plain flour, baking powder, cinnamon, and nutmeg.

3 In a medium mixing bowl, add the egg, brown sugar, almond milk, and apple sauce-mung bean mixture. Whisk until thoroughly combined.

4 Add the bean mixture to the flour mixture and stir until no streaks of dry ingredients remain. Gently fold in the diced apples until combined.

5 Line a 12-cup muffin pan with paper liners. Place 2 tablespoons of the mixture into each cup. Sprinkle the top of each muffin with 1 teaspoon of oats. Bake for 20–25 minutes until set, and a skewer inserted into the centre of the muffin comes out clean. Let rest for an hour before serving. Store in an airtight container for up to 2 days.

150g (5½oz) unsweetened apple sauce

85g (3oz) cooked mung beans

2 tbsp agave nectar

100g (3½oz) wholemeal flour

100g (3½oz) plain flour

2 tsp baking powder

1 tsp cinnamon

pinch of ground nutmeg

1 large egg

100g (3½oz) light brown sugar

80ml (3fl oz) unsweetened almond milk

1 medium Granny Smith apple, peeled, cored, and finely diced

20g (¾oz) rolled oats

Make it vegan

Substitute half a mashed banana for the egg.

Tropical Smoothie Bowl

The bright flavours of pineapple and mango are complemented by velvety white beans and banana in these beautiful, protein-rich bowls.

makes 2   **prep** 10 mins   **cook** none

1 Withhold a bit of mango, pineapple, and banana for the garnish. In a blender, add the remainder of the fruit, along with the honey, yogurt, and cannellini beans. Purée until completely smooth.

2 Divide the smoothie between 2 bowls, and garnish with toasted coconut, chia seeds, and the reserved mango, pineapple, and banana. Serve immediately.

175g (6oz) diced mango

200g (7oz) diced pineapple

1 banana, sliced

1 tbsp honey or agave nectar

200g (7oz) yogurt (see page 38)

85g (3oz) cooked cannellini beans

15g (½oz) toasted coconut, to garnish

2 tsp chia seeds, to garnish

Make it vegan

Use a vegan yogurt alternative, such as coconut yogurt (see page 38), rather than dairy yogurt.

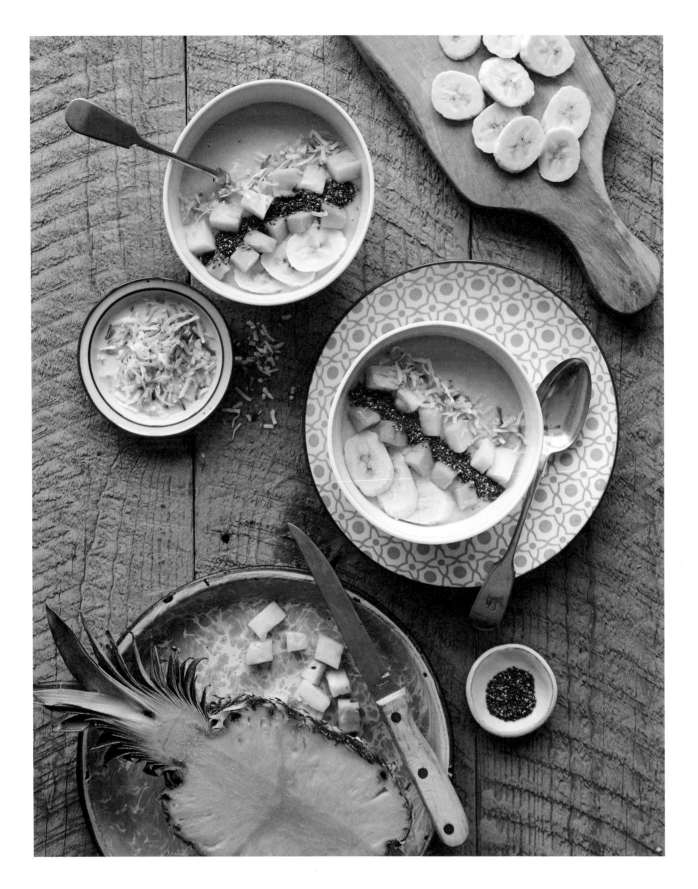

Wholemeal Pancakes with Apple and Cinnamon

Wholemeal flour gives these pancakes a rustic texture and nutty flavour, while apple adds sweetness and moisture.

makes 8   **prep** 15 mins   **cook** 6 minutes

1   In a large bowl, whisk together the wholemeal flour, baking powder, sugar, cinnamon, and salt. In a small bowl, beat together the egg and milk.

2   Make a well in the centre of the dry ingredients and pour in the milk mixture, whisking to combine. Once it is completely mixed, add the cooled, melted butter and whisk again. Gently fold in the grated apple.

3   In a large non-stick frying pan, melt a little butter over a medium heat. Spoon small amounts of batter into the hot pan, to create pancakes about 10cm (4in) across. Use the back of the spoon to smooth over the tops of the pancakes.

4   Cook for 3 minutes over a medium-low heat, until they look set around the edges. Carefully turn over and cook for another 2–3 minutes. Serve immediately with maple syrup and apple slices (if using), pan-fried in butter and finished with lemon juice.

150g (5½oz) wholemeal flour

1 tsp baking powder

1 tbsp sugar

½ tsp ground cinnamon

⅛ tsp fine sea salt

1 large egg

160ml (5½fl oz) whole milk

1 tbsp unsalted butter, melted and cooled, plus extra for frying

1 apple, peeled, cored, and finely grated

To serve

maple syrup

a few apple slices (optional)

lemon juice (optional)

Make it vegan

Mix together 1 tbsp chia seeds with 3 tbsp warm water, let it sit for 15 minutes and use this instead of the egg in step 1. Instead of dairy milk and butter, use soy milk and vegetable oil spread.

Wheat Berry Bircher Muesli Pots

Perfect for spring or summer, these bircher muesli pots replace the traditional oats with wheat berries that add a delicious nutty flavour and texture.

serves 4   **prep** 25 mins, plus overnight soaking and cooling   **cook** 30 mins

1 Place the wheat berries in a large bowl, cover with water, and leave to soak overnight or for up to 8 hours. Then drain well, rinse under running water, and drain again.

2 Place the wheat berries in a large saucepan, cover with plenty of water, and bring to the boil. Then reduce the heat to a simmer, cover, and cook for 30 minutes or until the wheat berries are tender. Remove from the heat, drain any remaining water, and leave to cool completely.

3 Meanwhile, wash the blueberries and place them in a separate bowl. Wash the strawberries and cut them into thin slices. Add them to the blueberries and toss to mix. Once cooled, place the wheat berries, yogurt, sunflower seeds, and honey in a large bowl. Mix until well combined.

4 Divide half the wheat berries and yogurt mixture equally between 4 serving bowls, glasses, or jars. Top with a layer of half of the strawberries and blueberries. Repeat the process adding one more layer of yogurt and fruit. Sprinkle over some sunflower seeds and add a drizzle of honey before serving.

120g (4¼oz) uncooked wheat berries

250g (9oz) blueberries

250g (9oz) strawberries, hulled

400g (14oz) yogurt (see page 38)

4 tbsp sunflower seeds, plus extra to serve

4 tbsp honey, plus extra to serve

Why not try...

Try adding raspberries and blackberries in place of the blueberries and strawberries.

Make it vegan

Substitute the dairy yogurt for a vegan alternative, such as coconut yogurt (see page 38), and use maple syrup or agave nectar instead of honey.

Snacks, Dips, and Light Bites

Sometimes you need a little something small to tide you over between main meals. These nutritious small bites are perfect for snacking, enjoying as appetizers, or serving as finger food to guests.

Raw Energy Bars

Mix and match the dried fruits and seeds in these healthy energy bars as you like, but keep the quantities the same.

makes 16 **prep** 10 minutes, plus 4 hours chilling time **cook** none

1 Put the dates and prunes in a heatproof bowl and cover with hot water. Leave to soak for 5 minutes. Put the hazelnuts in a food processor and pulse until they are broken up into pieces.

2 Drain the dates and prunes and loosely squeeze them dry, leaving them still damp. Place them in the food processor with the hazelnuts and add all the remaining ingredients.

3 Process the mixture until it is well combined, the nuts and seeds are in small pieces, and the mixture begins to form a ball. It will be very stiff, so you may need to scrape down the sides of the bowl and break it up occasionally with a spatula.

4 Turn out the mixture into a 23cm (9in) square baking tin, and use dampened hands to push it into an even layer. Use the back of a large metal spoon, dampened, to even out the surface of the mixture, then cover, and chill for at least 3–4 hours.

5 Turn out the mixture on to a board and cut into 16 equal-sized pieces. Wrap individually in baking parchment and store in an airtight container in the refrigerator until needed.

150g (5½oz) pitted Medjool dates, roughly chopped

100g (3½oz) pitted prunes, roughly chopped

60g (2oz) raw hazelnuts

60g (2oz) buckwheat flour

50g (1¾oz) raw sliced almonds

30g (1oz) unsweetened flaked coconut

60g (2oz) dried cherries, roughly chopped

30g (1oz) sprouted pumpkin seeds

30g (1oz) sprouted sunflower seeds

2 tbsp raw cacao powder

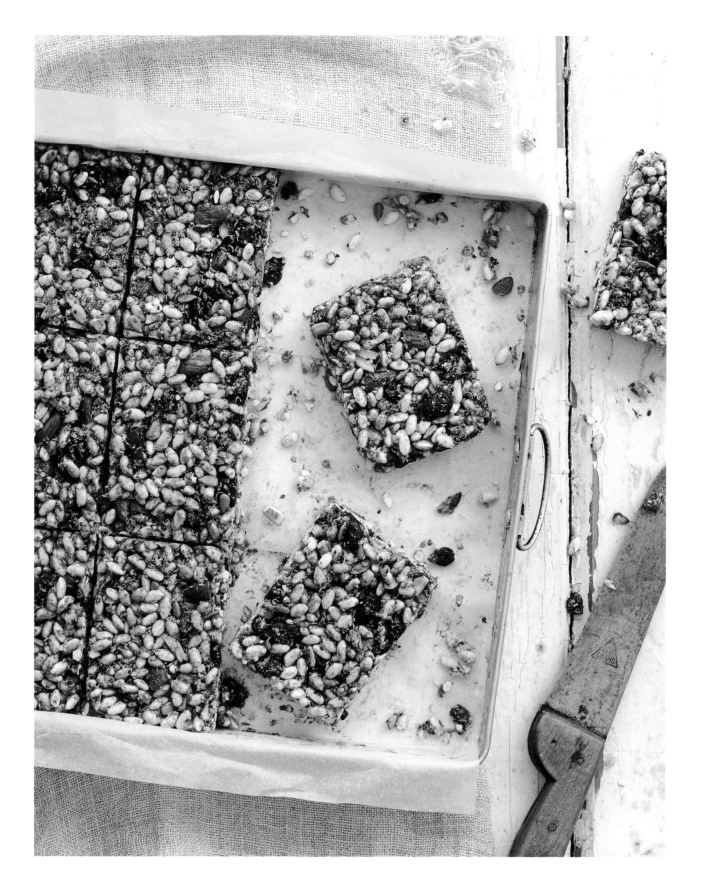

Cranberry, Orange and Chocolate Quinoa Bars

The perfect handy snack, these sweet, chewy and wholesome bars feel like a treat, but pack a big nutritional punch and will keep you full for hours.

makes 12 bars **prep** 20 mins, plus cooling **cook** 5 mins

1 Place the almonds, quinoa flakes, sunflower seeds, chia seeds, dried cranberries, puffed rice cereal, chocolate chips, and orange zest in a bowl. Mix well with a wooden spoon and set aside. Grease and line a 20 × 25cm (8 × 10in) baking tin with greaseproof paper.

2 Heat the oil, honey, and sugar in a saucepan over a medium heat. Cook, stirring occasionally, for about 5 minutes or until the sugar has melted and the mixture is bubbling. Set aside to cool for about 2 minutes.

3 Pour the cooled honey mixture into the dry ingredients. Mix using a wooden spoon until well incorporated, making sure the chocolate chips have melted and are evenly combined. Spoon the mixture into the prepared baking tin. Press down firmly with the back of a wooden spoon to make a roughly even layer.

4 Place the baking tin in the fridge for at least 4 hours, to allow the mixture to cool and harden. Remove from the fridge, turn out on to a chopping board, and cut into bars. These can be stored in an airtight container in the fridge for up to 5 days.

120g (4¼oz) almonds, roughly chopped

120g (4¼oz) quinoa flakes

35g (1¼oz) sunflower seeds

35g (1¼oz) chia seeds

100g (3½oz) dried cranberries

125g (4½oz) puffed rice cereal

50g (1¾oz) dark chocolate chips

grated zest of 2 large oranges

85ml (2¾fl oz) coconut oil

120ml (4fl oz) clear honey

35g (1oz) light brown sugar

Why not try...

Add walnuts instead of the almonds, pumpkin seeds instead of sunflower seeds, and raisins or chopped dates instead of the cranberries. In each case, use the same amount of the substitute ingredient as recommended in the recipe.

Make it vegan

Buy vegan dark chocolate chips, or replace the chocolate chips with extra dried cranberries. Instead of honey, use rice malt syrup.

Spicy Carrot Hummus

Harissa is a natural match for the sweetness of carrots and the tang of tahini in this hummus. Serve with crisp vegetables or seeded crackers.

serves 6 **prep** 20 mins **cook** 30 mins

1   Preheat the oven to 180°C (350°F). Peel the carrots and cut into 3cm (1in) chunks. Toss with 1 tablespoon of oil and arrange in a single layer on a baking tray. Roast for 25-30 minutes, until caramelized and tender. Remove from the oven and leave to cool.

2   In a food processor, combine the chickpeas and water and whizz briefly to combine. Add the tahini, lime juice, harissa, and roasted carrots. With the processor running on low, drizzle in the oil. Season with salt and pepper to taste, then pulse a few more times to combine. Serve immediately.

350g (12oz) carrots, ends trimmed, around 7-8 carrots

60ml (2fl oz) olive oil, plus 1 tbsp for roasting

350g (12oz) cooked chickpeas, peeled

1 tbsp water

1½ tbsp tahini

juice of 1 large lime

1 tbsp harissa paste

salt and freshly ground black pepper

Why not try...

Replace the chickpeas with an equal amount of cooked cannellini or navy beans.

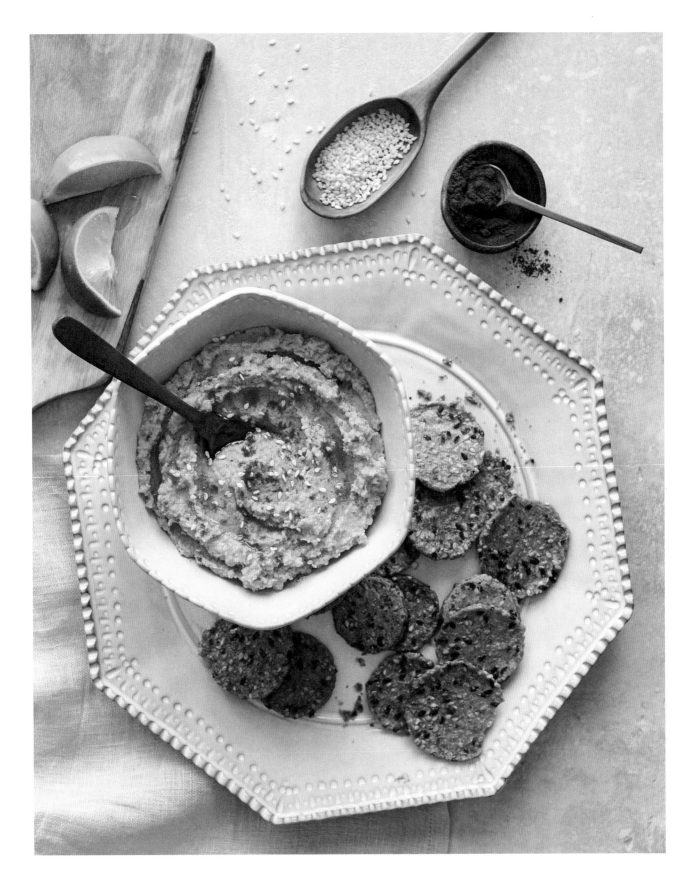

White Bean Butter with Radishes

Radishes with butter and salt are a classic French snack. Here, the butter is browned and blended with white beans to make a luxurious and creamy dip.

serves 4   **prep** 5 mins   **cook** 10 mins

1   In a small saucepan, melt the butter over a low heat. Cook until the butter takes on a light brown colour and nutty aroma, then remove from the heat.

2   In a food processor, combine the butter, cannellini beans, and garlic. Blend on high until smooth, adding water as needed to reach the desired consistency.

3   Transfer the dip to a small bowl and serve alongside radishes and a small dish of sea salt.

2 tbsp unsalted butter

175g (6oz) cooked cannellini beans

1 garlic clove

1 tsp water (optional)

1 bunch radishes, washed and tops removed

flaky sea salt

Make it vegan

Omit the butter for a more traditional white bean dip.

Adzuki Bean Summer Rolls with Peanut Sauce

Spiralized jicama replaces traditional rice noodles in these summer rolls. Adzuki beans complement the sweet mango and creamy avocado.

makes 16 **prep** 1 hr **cook** none

1 To make the peanut sauce, in a small bowl whisk together the peanut butter, lime juice, vinegar, water, and Sriracha until smooth. Set aside until ready to serve.

2 Cut the jicama into even chunks. Adjust a spiralizer to the thinnest blade and spiralize the jicama. Set out the jicama, mint, mango, onion, avocado, adzuki beans, and coriander on your worktop to prepare for filling the rolls.

3 Pour warm water into a shallow flan or pie dish. One at a time, submerge the rice paper wrapper into warm water for 30 seconds, or until pliable without tearing. Remove from the water and place onto a clean, flat, non-stick surface, such as a plastic or ceramic cutting board.

4 Arrange the desired amount of mint leaves, mango, red onion, avocado, adzuki beans, coriander, and spiralized jicama in the centre of the wrapper, working quickly so that it doesn't dry out. Do not overstuff the wrapper, or it will tear. Fold the bottom edge over the filling, and press to seal. Then fold the sides towards the centre, tucking in the filling. Roll gently and seal firmly.

5 Repeat to use all the remaining ingredients. Serve with peanut sauce on the side. Store in the fridge for 2–3 days, individually wrapped so they do not stick together.

125g (4½oz) smooth peanut butter

juice of 1 lime

1 tbsp rice wine vinegar

80ml (3fl oz) water

½ tsp Sriracha

1 small jicama, peeled (if you can't find jicama, try using water chestnuts or Jerusalem artichokes)

25g (1oz) mint leaves

1 mango, peeled, stoned, and cut into 1cm (½in) slices

1 small red onion, julienned

1 avocado, pitted and cut into 5mm (¼in) slices

325g (11oz) cooked adzuki beans

60g (2oz) coriander leaves

1 packet of spring roll rice paper wrappers

Make it with fish

Horizontally slice 1 cooked king prawn for each roll, and place atop the mint during assembly.

Shirataki and Prawn Summer Rolls

These light and tasty rolls are stuffed with shirataki noodles, prawns and fresh herbs, but they can take a variety of fillings. Use vibrant, crisp vegetables and mix and match as you prefer.

makes 8 rolls   **prep** 30 mins   **cook** none

1   To make the dipping sauce: in a small saucepan, heat the sugar and 2 tablespoons water over a medium heat, whisking frequently, until the sugar has dissolved. Remove from the heat and leave to cool. Then add the remaining ingredients and whisk to combine.

2   Fill a large bowl with warm water. Fully submerge 1 rice paper wrapper for 10 to 15 seconds until it just starts to soften. Shake any excess water from it, and lay it flat on a clean work surface.

3   Take 2 prawn halves and lay them pink-side down along the centre of the wrapper. Top the prawn with a few leaves of mint, basil, and coriander. Then add a little of the shirataki noodles, a few julienned carrots and spring onions, and a few pea shoots, leaving the edges of the wrapper free. Finish with 2 more prawn halves, pink-side up.

4   The wrapper should be fully softened and pliable by now, but not too delicate. Wrap the nearest side to you up over the filling, tuck the outside edges up over the filling, and roll the wrapper away from you, tucking as you go, to fully encase the filling. Place on a plate, cover with damp kitchen paper, and refrigerate. Repeat steps 2 to 4 to make all 8 rolls, continuing to chill them as you go.

5   After assembling all 8 rolls, serve immediately with the dipping sauce on the side.

8 × 15cm (6in) rice paper wrappers

16 large, cooked prawns, halved horizontally

small handful of coriander leaves

small handful of mint leaves

small handful of Thai basil leaves

2 × 200g packet shirataki noodles, drained, rinsed, and dried

1 large carrot, julienned

4 spring onions, julienned

small handful of pea shoots

for the dipping sauce

2 tbsp sugar

1½ tbsp fish sauce

1 tbsp rice wine vinegar

juice of 1 lime

½ garlic clove, crushed

pinch of red pepper flakes

Make it vegan

These summer rolls will taste just as great without prawns. But you could also add extra vegetables or slices of firm tofu if you wish.

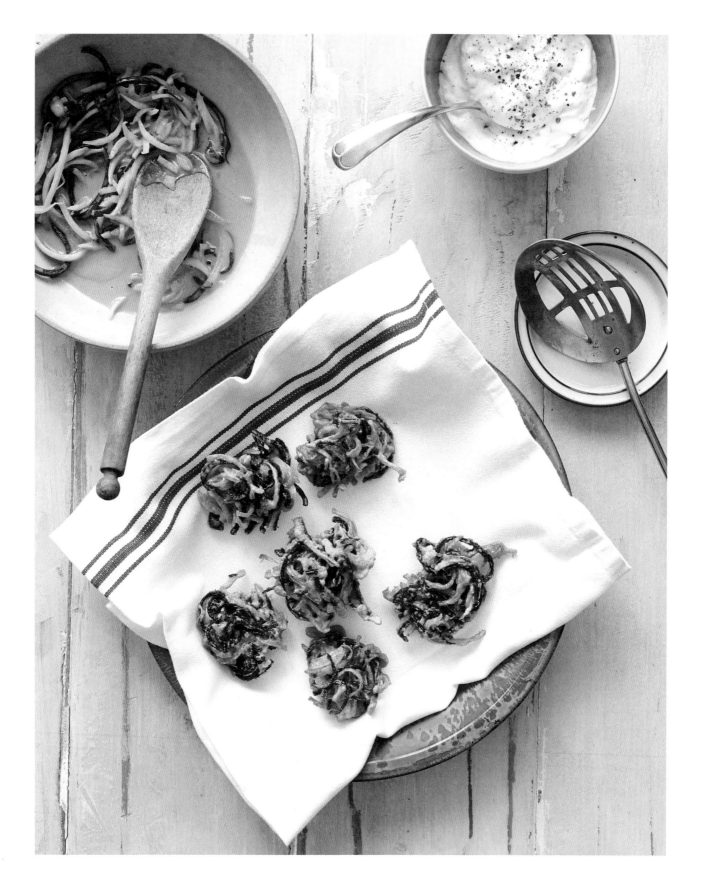

Spiralized Beetroot and Onion Bhajis

These crispy Indian fritters can be eaten as an appetizer or snack. The spiralized beetroot adds a vivid pink colour.

serves 12   **prep** 15 mins   **cook** 15 mins

1 In a large flameproof casserole or heavy-based saucepan, heat the canola oil over a medium-low heat. Measuring with a deep frying thermometer, bring to 180°C (350°F).

2 Meanwhile, to make the cucumber sauce, in a small bowl stir together the yogurt and cucumber.

3 Adjust a spiralizer to the thinnest blade and spiralize the onion and beetroot. With kitchen scissors, trim into 3cm (1in) lengths.

4 In a large mixing bowl, whisk together the turmeric, salt, chickpea flour, and water. Gradually add water to reach the consistency of pancake batter. Add the beetroot and onion and toss to combine.

5 With your hands, gather 2 tablespoons of the bhaji mixture and carefully drop into the oil. Fry for 4 minutes, or until golden and crispy, rotating once. Place on a plate lined with kitchen paper and repeat with the remaining batter. Serve immediately with the cucumber sauce.

1 litre (1¾ pints) canola oil

200g (7oz) plain Greek-style yogurt

1 small cucumber, peeled and grated

1 large onion, peeled

1 large beetroot, peeled

pinch of turmeric

½ tsp salt

75g (2½oz) chickpea flour

120ml (4fl oz) water

Make it vegan

Replace the Greek-style yogurt in the sauce with the same quantity of coconut milk yogurt (see page 38).

Quinoa and Moth Bean Dolmades

Distinctive dill and mint combine with the textures of currants and pine nuts in these stuffed vine leaves, whose flavours develop over time for a delicious make-ahead lunch.

makes 24   **prep** 30 mins   **cook** 1 hr

1 Preheat the oven to 180°C (350°F). Lightly grease a 23 × 30cm (9 × 12in) glass or ceramic baking dish. Fill a large bowl with warm water. Soak the vine leaves for 2–3 minutes until pliable. Drain in a colander. Cover the colander with a wet towel, so they remain moist during assembly.

2 To make the filling, in a large mixing bowl combine the quinoa, mint, dill, parsley, currants, pine nuts, 1 tablespoon of oil, 1 tablespoon of lemon juice, and the cooked moth beans (or lentils). Season with salt and pepper.

3 To assemble the dolmades, place one vine leaf on a clean, flat work surface, vein-side up, and cut off the stem. Place 1 heaped tablespoon of filling in the centre, towards the bottom of the leaf. Fold the sides over the filling and roll tightly from stem to tip. Place seam-side down in the baking dish. Repeat with the remaining leaves, arranging snugly.

4 Pour the stock over the dolmades and drizzle over the remaining 1 tablespoon of oil and 2 tablespoons of lemon juice.

5 Cover the baking dish with foil and bake for 20–30 minutes until all the liquid has absorbed and the dolmades are moist and steaming. Serve immediately or leave to cool and store in an airtight container in the fridge for up to 2 days.

225g (8oz) jar of vine leaves, minimum 24 leaves

140g (5oz) cooked quinoa

1½ tbsp chopped mint leaves

1½ tbsp chopped dill

1½ tbsp chopped flat-leaf parsley

45g (1½oz) dried currants

30g (1oz) toasted pine nuts

2 tbsp olive oil

3 tbsp lemon juice

300g (10oz) cooked moth beans, or black lentils

salt and freshly ground black pepper

240ml (8fl oz) vegetable stock

Why not try...

For a tangier bite, sprinkle 45g (1½oz) of finely crumbled feta cheese or nut cheese into the quinoa filling before rolling the dolmades.

Make it with meat

Stir in 45g (1½oz) cooked minced lamb or beef with the quinoa filling.

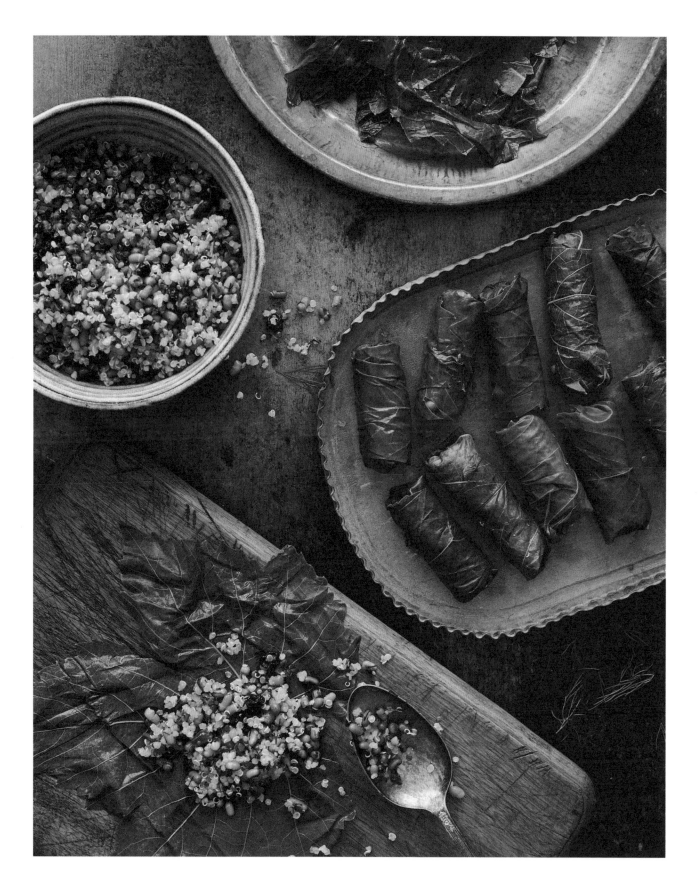

Masala Chickpea Nachos

This hybrid recipe combines the warm spices of Indian cuisine with the cheesy crunch of Tex-Mex nachos.

serves 6   **prep** 40 mins   **cook** 20 mins

1 To make the coriander-mint sauce, in a blender combine two-thirds of the coriander with the mint, lemon juice, ginger, and water. Purée until smooth. Season with salt and pepper. Transfer to an airtight container and set aside.

2 Preheat the oven to 200°C (400°F). Line a baking tray with foil. Toss the chickpeas with the curry powder, garam masala, and oil. Spread in an even layer on the baking tray and bake for 10 minutes, or until just crispy and warmed through. Transfer to a bowl and wipe the baking tray.

3 Break each poppadom into quarters and arrange in a single layer on the baking tray. Sprinkle half the mozzarella over the poppadoms and top with the chickpea mixture. Then top with the remaining mozzarella and bake for 10–12 minutes, until the mozzarella melts and the poppadoms are lightly brown.

4 Meanwhile, in a small saucepan, heat the mango chutney with 1 tablespoon of water. Cook for 2–3 minutes until thin and warmed through.

5 To finish the assembly, sprinkle the onion over the melted cheese and drizzle mango chutney sauce over the top. Dollop the coriander-mint sauce across the nachos. Chop the remaining coriander and sprinkle over the nachos. Garnish with lime wedges and serve immediately, directly from the tray.

125g (4½oz) coriander leaves

30g (1oz) mint leaves

2 tbsp lemon juice

¼ tsp ground ginger

80ml (3fl oz) cold water

salt and freshly ground black pepper

350g (12oz) cooked chickpeas

1 tsp curry powder

1 tsp garam masala

1 tbsp vegetable oil

10 poppadoms, cooked according to instructions

225g (8oz) grated mozzarella cheese

125g (4½oz) mango chutney

30g (1oz) diced red onion

1 large lime, cut into 6 wedges

Make it vegan

Use a soy mozzarella-style cheese alternative or nut cheese (see page 37) instead of mozzarella.

Make it with meat

Add 125g (4½oz) cooked chopped chicken with the chickpeas in step 3.

Chickpea Flour Socca with Herb and Green Olive Salad

Socca – a chickpea flour pancake – hails from the south of France. Its mild, nutty flavour is the perfect canvas for the fresh herbs and flavours of the rocket salad.

serves 2   **prep** 5 mins, plus 1 hr for batter to rest   **cook** 15 mins

1   To make the batter, in a medium mixing bowl add the chickpea flour, paprika, garlic powder, salt, 2 tablespoons oil, and water. Whisk to combine. Let rest at room temperature for 1 hour.

2   With the rack in the middle of the oven, place two 20cm (8in) cast-iron or ovenproof frying pans in the oven and preheat to 230°C (450°F). (The pans will heat up with the oven.)

3   When the frying pans are heated, carefully remove and swirl 1½ teaspoons oil around in each. Pour half the batter into each and return to the oven. Bake for 8 minutes. Then turn the grill onto a low setting and cook for an additional 2 minutes. Remove and let rest for 1–2 minutes.

4   Meanwhile, to make the herb and olive salad, toss together the rocket, parsley, basil, olives, and lemon juice. Place each socca on a serving plate and top with an equal amount of salad. Serve immediately.

100g (3½oz) chickpea flour

1 tsp smoked paprika

⅛ tsp garlic powder

pinch of salt

3 tbsp olive oil

240ml (8fl oz) water

45g (1½oz) rocket leaves

10g (¼oz) flat-leaf parsley

5g (⅛oz) basil leaves

45g (1½oz) pitted green olives, halved

juice of 1 lemon

Make it with meat

To turn this into a main meal, top the salad with sliced, grilled steak.

Savoury Green Pancakes with Feta and Sprout Salad

This recipe is inspired by okonomiyaki, a Japanese street food. Prepare the sprout salad with the herbs of your choice.

makes 4 **prep** 10 minutes **cook** 15 mins

1 In a large bowl, whisk together the flour and baking powder with a pinch of salt and pepper. Add the egg and then the vegetable stock, a little at a time, whisking constantly to produce a smooth, thick batter. Add the cabbage, mung beans, spring onions, and dill, and mix until completely combined.

2 In a non-stick frying pan, heat a bit of butter and olive oil over a medium heat until the butter sizzles. Scoop one-quarter of the batter into the pan and use a spatula to press it into a firm, even pancake. Cook over a medium-low heat for 3–4 minutes.

3 When the underside is brown and crispy, slide the pancake on to a plate. Add more butter and oil to the pan and carefully flip the pancake back into the pan to cook the other side for 3–4 minutes. Remove from the pan and keep the pancake warm while you cook 3 more, using the same process.

4 Toss the sprouts with the herbs, dress with the lemon juice and the 1 tbsp of olive oil, and season with salt and pepper. Gently crumble in the feta cheese. Serve the pancakes immediately, topped with the sprout salad.

60g (2oz) plain flour

¼ tsp baking powder

salt and freshly ground black pepper

1 large egg, lightly beaten

85ml (3fl oz) vegetable stock

100g (3½oz) savoy cabbage, coarse stalks removed, shredded

100g (3½oz) sprouted mung beans

4 spring onions, finely sliced

2 tbsp finely chopped dill fronds

unsalted butter, for frying

1 tbsp olive oil, plus extra for frying

60g (2oz) mixed mustard, red clover, and alfalfa sprouts

handful of mixed herbs, chopped

½ tbsp lemon juice

100g (3½oz) feta cheese

Make it vegan

Create a flax egg by mixing 1 tbsp flax seeds with 3 tbsp warm water and letting it sit for 15 minutes. Add this instead of the egg in step 1. Simply omit the feta or use a nut cheese (see page 37) instead.

Burgers, Tacos, and Wraps

Reducing your meat intake doesn't mean you have to stop eating burgers! Enjoy a variety of vegetarian burger recipes, as well as new ways to make tacos, quesadillas, and wraps.

Mung Bean Burgers with Red Curry Aioli

Mung beans provide this textured veggie burger with great bite and a lovely green colour.

serves 6   **prep** 25 mins   **cook** 25 mins

1 Preheat the oven to 190°C (375°F). Line a baking sheet with baking parchment or spray with cooking spray. In a large mixing bowl, combine the shallot, garlic, mung beans, ground coriander, chillies, coriander leaves, and mint. With a pastry cutter or the back of a fork, lightly mash the mixture, allowing about half the mung beans to remain intact.

2 Add the eggs and stir to mix thoroughly. Gently fold in the breadcrumbs and season with salt and pepper.

3 Divide the mung bean mixture into 6 equal portions. Use a measuring cup to place a rounded portion onto the baking sheet and lightly flatten it to make a burger. Repeat to make 6 in total. Bake for 10 minutes on each side, carefully turning in between.

4 Meanwhile, to make the red curry aioli, in a small mixing bowl whisk together the yogurt and red curry paste. Season with salt and pepper to taste.

5 To assemble, spread the curry aioli on the bottom half of the bun or inside of the pitta and add the burger. Repeat for the remaining burgers and serve immediately.

1 shallot, finely chopped

1 garlic clove, finely chopped

350g (12oz) cooked mung beans

¼ tsp ground coriander

pinch of crushed dried chillies

2 tbsp chopped coriander leaves

1 tbsp chopped mint leaves

2 large eggs, beaten

20g (¾oz) panko breadcrumbs

salt and freshly ground black pepper

100g (3½oz) plain Greek-style yogurt

½ tbsp red curry paste

6 hamburger buns or small pittas

Why not try...

For a double dose of legumes and texture, top your burger with alfalfa sprouts.

Make it vegan

Mix 2 tablespoons flax seeds with 6 tablespoons water and let it sit for 15 minutes to replace the eggs. Replace the Greek yogurt with coconut yogurt (see page 38).

Black-eyed Bean Sliders with Pico de Gallo

The pico de gallo adds a wonderful texture and moisture to these creamy black-eyed bean burgers.

serves 8   **prep** 30 mins   **cook** 20 mins

1   Preheat the oven to 150°C (300°F). In a large non-stick frying pan, heat the oil over a medium-low heat until shimmering. Add one of the onions and cook for 2 minutes, or until soft. Add the garlic and half the jalapeño. Cook for 2 minutes. Transfer to a large mixing bowl and set aside. Set aside the frying pan, leaving any residual oil in the pan.

2   Add the chipotle chilli powder, cumin, black-eyed beans, eggs, and breadcrumbs to the vegetable mixture. With a potato masher, mix to combine and break up the beans slightly.

3   Return the frying pan to the stove and heat over a medium heat. Divide the mixture into 8 equal portions and use your hands to form into patties. In batches, cook for 3–4 minutes on each side, pressing lightly with a spatula to sear. Transfer the patties to a baking sheet. Repeat to use all the mixture, adding ½ teaspoon oil to the frying pan between batches. Transfer the baking sheet to the oven and bake for 8–10 minutes until cooked through.

4   Meanwhile, to make the pico de gallo, in a small bowl combine the tomato, the remaining diced onion, remaining jalapeño, chopped coriander, and lime juice. To assemble, place each burger on a slider bun and top with 1 tablespoon of pico de gallo. Serve immediately.

1 tbsp plus 1 tsp olive oil

2 small onions, diced

1 garlic clove, finely chopped

2 small jalapeños, deseeded and diced, about 3 tbsp in total

½ tsp chipotle chilli powder

2½ tsp ground cumin

450g (1lb) cooked black-eyed beans

2 large eggs, beaten

20g (¾oz) panko breadcrumbs

1 large tomato, deseeded and diced

10g (¼oz) chopped coriander leaves

juice of 1 large lime

8 slider-sized burger buns

Why not try...

Give these sliders more crunch by topping with shredded green or red cabbage.

Make it with meat

To add smokiness, finely dice 1 bacon rasher and cook along with the garlic and jalapeño in step 1.

Bean Burgers with Raw Cashew Mayo

These filling burgers can be made with any type of firm legume, such as lentils, haricot beans or chickpeas.

serves 4   **prep** 15 mins, plus chilling   **cook** 1 hr

1   Place the beans in a saucepan of cold water and bring to the boil. Reduce the heat to a simmer and cook for 35–40 minutes until soft. Drain and rinse the beans; set aside to cool.

2   In a non-stick frying pan, heat 2 tablespoons of the oil over a medium heat. Add the mushrooms and cook for 5–7 minutes, until they are cooked through. Set aside to cool.

3   Put the beans, mushrooms, breadcrumbs, onion, parsley, Worcestershire sauce, and egg into a food processor and season with salt and pepper. Pulse the mixture until it is just mixed but still has some texture. With damp hands, shape the mixture into 4 patties and chill, covered, for 1 hour.

4   To make the cashew mayo, drain the cashews and place them in a food processor with the lemon juice, olive oil, garlic, and 5–6 tbsp of water. Process until smooth, then chill until needed.

5   In a large non-stick frying pan, heat the remaining 2 tbsp of oil over a medium heat. Cook the burger patties for 3–4 minutes on each side, until well browned and cooked through. Serve immediately on toasted buns, topped with avocado and tomato slices, alfalfa sprouts, and the cashew mayo.

450g (1lb) mixed beans

4 tbsp canola oil

60g (2oz) chestnut mushrooms, finely chopped

150g (5½oz) fresh white breadcrumbs

½ small onion, finely grated

2 tbsp finely chopped flat-leaf parsley leaves

2 tsp Worcestershire sauce

1 large egg, lightly beaten

salt and freshly ground pepper

120g (4¼oz) raw cashews, soaked for 3 hours

2 tbsp lemon juice

1 tbsp olive oil

1 small garlic clove, crushed

To serve

4 hamburger buns, toasted

sliced avocado and tomato

handful of alfalfa sprouts

Make it vegan

Mix 1 tbsp of flax seeds with 3 tbsp water and let it sit for 15 minutes to replace the egg.

Seeded Beetroot and Buckwheat Burgers

These hearty and earthy vegetarian burgers combine the sweetness of beetroot and the nutty texture of seeds with wholesome buckwheat. You won't miss the meat with these!

serves 4 **prep** 15 mins, plus soaking and chilling **cook** 30 mins

1 Place the buckwheat in a large bowl and cover with water. Cover the bowl with a kitchen towel and leave to soak for at least 8 hours or for up to 12 hours. Then drain and rinse under running water.

2 Place the beetroot, carrots, and onions in a food processor and pulse for 1–2 minutes to combine. Then add the buckwheat, eggs, oatmeal, and salt and pulse until just incorporated.

3 Add 50g (1¾oz) of the sunflower seeds to the mixture, pulse to combine, and transfer to a large bowl. Add the remaining sunflower seeds and stir to combine. Chill in the fridge for 30 minutes. Divide the mixture into 4 equal portions, then shape each portion into a 9cm (4in) wide and 2cm (¾in) thick burger patty.

4 Heat the oil in a non-stick frying pan over a medium-high heat. Add the patties, once the oil is hot, and fry for about 5 minutes on each side or until firm and lightly coloured. Do this in batches to avoid overcrowding the pan. Remove from the heat and drain on a plate lined with kitchen paper. Serve with burger buns, mayonnaise, chips, and a green salad.

60g (2oz) uncooked buckwheat

125g (4½oz) beetroot, unpeeled and roughly chopped

85g (3oz) carrot, unpeeled and roughly chopped

30g (1oz) spring onions, trimmed and finely chopped

2 eggs

60g (2oz) oatmeal

½ tsp salt

60g (2oz) sunflower seeds

2–3 tbsp vegetable oil

Why not try...

Use pumpkin seeds in place of the sunflower seeds.

Make it vegan

Substitute the eggs with 2 tbsp flax seeds mixed with 6 tbsp water. Let the mixture sit for 15 minutes before you use it in step 2.

Veggie Burger with Spelt

These vegetarian burgers get their intense flavour from the super-absorbent spelt grain. Roasting the vegetables before they are added to the burgers helps retain more of their flavour and keeps the unnecessary moisture out.

serves 6 **prep** 15 mins, plus overnight soaking and chilling **cook** 1 hr

1   Place the spelt in a bowl, cover with water, and leave to soak overnight. Then drain well and rinse under running water. Place the spelt in a lidded saucepan. Pour over 240ml (8fl oz) of water and bring to the boil. Then reduce the heat to a simmer, cover, and cook for 50 minutes. Remove from the heat and set aside to cool.

2   Preheat the oven to 220°C (425°F/Gas 7). Spread out the mushrooms on a lined baking sheet and toss with 2 teaspoons of the tamari sauce. Spread out the beetroots, carrots, and beans on a separate sheet. Season with salt and pepper and toss with the oil. Place the sheets in the oven and bake for about 15 minutes. Then remove from the heat and lightly toss the vegetables and mushrooms. Return to the oven, rotating the positions of the sheets. Bake for a further 10 minutes or until the vegetables and beans are crisp and the mushrooms have lost most of their moisture. Remove from the heat and leave to cool.

3   Place the ground almonds, breadcrumbs, cooled vegetables, and remaining tamari in a food processor and pulse until just combined. Add the mustard, mayonnaise, spring onions, garlic, and eggs to the mixture. Season to taste with pepper and pulse to combine. Then add the spelt and tempeh and pulse lightly until just mixed, but still retaining some texture. Transfer the mixture to a large bowl, cover, and chill in the fridge for about 1 hour.

4   Set the grill or griddle pan at its medium-low setting. Divide the mixture into 6 equal portions and form each into a 2.5cm- (1in-) thick patty. Grill the patties for about 5 minutes on each side, until crisp on the outside. Remove from the heat. Serve hot in burger buns, topped with avocado, tomato, and onion slices.

40g (1½oz) uncooked spelt grains (available from health food stores)

140g (5oz) shiitake mushrooms, sliced

3 tsp tamari or low-sodium soy sauce

1 large beetroot, about 100g (3½oz), grated

2 large carrots, about 100g (3½oz), grated

400g can kidney beans, drained

salt and freshly ground black pepper

1–2 tbsp olive oil

50g (1¾oz) ground almonds

40g (1½oz) panko breadcrumbs

2 tbsp spicy Dijon mustard

2 tbsp mayonnaise

2 spring onions, sliced

2 garlic cloves, pressed

2 large eggs

115g (4oz) tempeh, crumbled

For serving

6 burger buns

1 avocado, pitted and sliced

1 large tomato, sliced into rounds

1 large red onion, sliced into rounds

Make it vegan

Combine 2 tbsp flax seeds with 6 tbsp warm water and let it sit for 15 minutes. Use this instead of the eggs in step 3. Substitute a vegan mayonnaise (see page 39) too.

Pinto Bean and Spiralized Sweet Potato Quesadilla

This quesadilla is a great combination of heat from the jalapeño and sweetness from the potato. Spiralizing the sweet potato adds texture to this Mexican snack.

makes 4   **prep** 20 mins   **cook** 40 mins

1 With the medium blade of a spiralizer, spiralize the sweet potato.

2 In a medium frying pan, heat the oil over a medium-low heat until shimmering. Add the jalapeño and cook for 3 minutes, or until tender but not brown. Add the sweet potato and cook for 7 minutes, or until just al dente.

3 To assemble, place 1 tortilla on a clean, flat surface. Sprinkle about 30g (1oz) Cheddar on the lower half of the tortilla. Top with quarter of the pinto beans and quarter of the sweet potato. Add 2 tablespoons of onion and 2 tablespoons of coriander. Top with about another 30g (1oz) Cheddar, then fold over the top of the tortilla to create a semicircle. Repeat to make 4 quesadillas in total.

4 Heat a non-stick frying pan over a medium heat. Add 1 quesadilla and cook for 4 minutes. Carefully turn, cover, and cook for another 4 minutes, until the tortilla is golden and the cheese melted. Repeat for the remaining 3 quesadillas.

5 Cut each quesadilla into 4 sections. Serve immediately with soured cream on the side.

1 small sweet potato, peeled

2 tbsp vegetable oil

1 jalapeño, deseeded and diced

4 large flour tortillas

225g (8oz) finely grated mature Cheddar cheese

200g (7oz) cooked pinto or borlotti beans

45g (1½oz) chopped spring onion

15g (½oz) chopped coriander leaves

soured cream, to serve

Make it with meat

Layer 30g (1oz) cooked, chopped chicken or pork on top of the sweet potato in step 3.

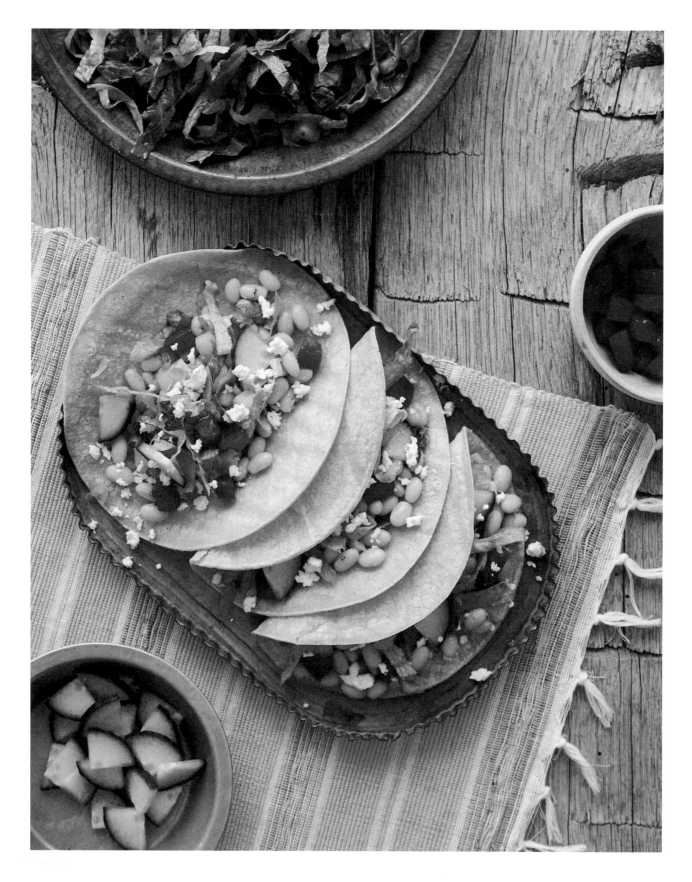

Greek White Bean Tacos

This twist on the traditional taco features ingredients typically found in a Greek salad. Romaine lettuce and cucumber add freshness and crunch to the creamy white beans and feta.

makes 8   **prep** 25 mins   **cook** 1 hr

1 In a small casserole or saucepan, heat the oil over a medium-low heat. Add the garlic and cook for 1–2 minutes until soft but not brown. Add the haricot beans, lemon zest and juice, and stock.

2 Bring to a simmer then reduce the heat to low and cook, covered, for 5–6 minutes, until the stock has been absorbed. Stir in the oregano. Season with salt and pepper to taste.

3 To assemble, spread 1 tablespoon of yogurt on a tortilla. Divide the bean mixture into 8 portions and add one portion to the tortilla. Top with a portion of lettuce, then tomato, and cucumber. Sprinkle the feta on top. Repeat with the remaining 7 tortillas, fold, and serve immediately.

2 tbsp olive oil

1 garlic clove, crushed

450g (1lb) cooked haricot beans

zest and juice of 1 large lemon

60ml (2fl oz) vegetable stock

1 tbsp chopped oregano

salt and freshly ground black pepper

100g (3½oz) plain Greek-style yogurt

8 small corn or flour tortillas

85g (3oz) shredded romaine lettuce

350g (12oz) diced plum tomatoes

140g (5oz) diced cucumber

115g (4oz) feta cheese, crumbled

Make it with meat

Add 75g (2½oz) cooked, chopped prawns or chicken along with the beans in step 1.

Quinoa Falafel with Mint Yogurt Sauce

The addition of quinoa to the traditional falafel gives them an added wholegrain goodness and a unique flavour and texture. It is paired here with a fresh and light yogurt sauce to complement the earthy spices.

serves 4   **prep** 15 mins, plus chilling   **cook** 45 mins

1 Rinse the quinoa under running water, place in a large saucepan, and cover with 170ml (6fl oz) of water. Place the pan over a medium heat and bring to a simmer. Cook the quinoa for 15 minutes or until almost all the water has been absorbed. Remove from the heat, drain any remaining water, and set aside.

2 Place the quinoa, egg, garlic, cumin, salt, and 350g (12oz) of the chickpeas in a food processor. Pulse until well combined. Add the coriander and the remaining chickpeas and pulse lightly for 1 minute, until the chickpeas have broken down but still retain some of their texture. Transfer the mixture to a large bowl and chill in the fridge for 30 minutes.

3 Preheat the oven to 200°C (400°F/Gas 6). Grease and line a baking sheet with greaseproof paper. Divide the falafel mixture into eight equal portions. On a lightly floured surface, roll each portion into a smooth ball and press down lightly to form patty-like shapes.

4 Brush the falafel with a little oil on both sides and place on the baking sheet. Bake in the oven for 20 minutes or until the falafel are well browned and crispy on the outside. Remove from the heat.

5 For the sauce, place all the ingredients in a bowl and mix well. Serve the falafel and mint yogurt sauce with pitta breads and a green salad, if liked.

60g (2oz) uncooked quinoa

1 egg

2 garlic cloves

1 tbsp cumin

¼ tsp salt

2 × 400g cans chickpeas, drained

4 tbsp chopped coriander leaves

1 tbsp plain flour, for dusting

1–2 tbsp olive oil, plus extra for greasing

For the sauce

150g (5½oz) Greek yogurt

4 tbsp chopped mint leaves

juice of 1 lemon

Make it vegan

Reserve 3 tbsp aquafaba before you drain the chickpeas. Add this instead of the egg in step 2. Substitute coconut yogurt (see page 38) for the sauce.

Baked Falafel with Pickled Red Onions

For a healthier version of the Middle Eastern street snack, this falafel is oven-baked instead of fried. Pickled onions and sambal oelek are the perfect tangy-sweet and spicy condiments.

serves 16 **prep** 30 mins, plus 3 hrs to chill **cook** 40 mins

1 To make the pickled red onions, in a medium saucepan bring the apple cider vinegar, red wine vinegar, sugar, and salt to the boil over a medium heat. Stir until the sugar and salt dissolve. Remove from the heat and stir in the red onion. Leave to cool completely at room temperature, stirring occasionally. Pour into a glass jar and secure with a lid. Refrigerate for 3 hours or overnight.

2 Preheat the oven to 200°C (400°F). In a food processor, combine the garlic, chickpeas, bicarbonate of soda, ground coriander, cumin, chillies, parsley, chopped coriander, and lemon zest and juice. Pulse until combined but not smooth.

3 Transfer the chickpea mixture to a medium mixing bowl and fold in the chickpea flour. Drizzle oil over and stir once more until it holds together. Season with salt and pepper to taste.

4 Portion out approximately 2 tablespoons of chickpea mixture and roll into a ball with your hands. Place on a baking tray and repeat with the remaining mixture. With a spatula, slightly flatten each one. Bake for 10 minutes, turn over, and bake for an additional 10 minutes. Serve immediately with the pickled red onions and sambal oelek on the side.

240ml (8fl oz) apple cider vinegar

120ml (4fl oz) red wine vinegar

2 tbsp sugar

1 tsp salt

1 large red onion, thinly sliced

1 garlic clove

350g (12oz) cooked chickpeas

½ tsp bicarbonate of soda

½ tsp ground coriander

½ tsp ground cumin

pinch of crushed dried chillies

1 bunch of curly parsley, chopped

20g (¾oz) finely chopped coriander leaves

zest and juice of 1 lemon

20g (¾oz) chickpea flour

1 tbsp olive oil

salt and freshly ground black pepper

75g (2½oz) sambal oelek

Why not try...

If you'd rather skip the heat, serve with tzatziki sauce instead of spicy sambal.

Make it with meat

Add 225g (8oz) raw minced lamb along with the olive oil in step 3.

Salads

Perfect to enjoy as a filling lunch or as a delicious side to your main meal, these fresh, bright salads will make it easy to eat your five a day.

Thai Noodle Salad

Making your own quick pickles is easy, and their refreshing, sharp flavours can really finish a dish. Lotus root is beautiful, but normal radishes work just as well.

serves 6 **prep** 30 mins, plus pickling **cook** none

1 To make the pickled lotus: soak the lotus root in cold water for 20 to 30 minutes. Drain, then blanch in boiling water for 1 to 2 minutes. Drain and refresh under cold water, then stack the slices in a small glass jar. Whisk together the rice wine vinegar, sugar, and salt until the sugar has dissolved. Pour the vinegar mixture over the lotus root, cover, and refrigerate for at least 1 day and up to 5 days before using.

2 To make the dressing: whisk together all the ingredients, along with 2 tablespoons water, until the sugar has dissolved.

3 Place the noodles in a heatproof bowl and cover with boiling water. Soak for 15 minutes until soft, and snip with kitchen scissors to make a more manageable length to eat. Drain, rinse well under cold water, and set aside to cool and drain completely.

4 In a large bowl, combine the cooled noodles with the finely sliced vegetables, dried shrimp, and most of the chopped herbs and peanuts. Add the dressing and toss very well until the dressing is completely incorporated.

5 Heap the salad into the middle of a serving bowl and scatter with the reserved herbs and peanuts. Top with the pickled lotus root and serve immediately with any extra dressing and lotus root on the side.

225g (8oz) dried glass noodles

225g (8oz) green papaya or green mango, julienned

2 carrots, julienned

½ small red onion, very finely sliced

2 under-ripe tomatoes, halved and cut into very thin wedges

2 tbsp dried shrimp, very finely chopped or crushed with a mortar and pestle

handful of mint leaves, roughly chopped

handful of coriander leaves, roughly chopped

2 tbsp salted peanuts, roughly chopped

For the pickled lotus

1 lotus root, peeled and thinly sliced, about 100g (3½oz) in total

120ml (4fl oz) rice wine vinegar

50g (1¾ oz) sugar

1 tsp fine sea salt

For the dressing

4 tsp sugar

4 tbsp lime juice

2 tbsp fish sauce

2 tbsp rice wine vinegar

1 garlic clove, crushed

Make it vegan

Simply omit the dried shrimp, and use a vegan fish sauce or soy sauce in the dressing in place of fish sauce.

Make it with meat

Add 180g cooked, chopped chicken with the noodles, dried shrimp, herbs and peanuts in step 4.

Rainbow Bowl with Sesame and Ginger Dressing

To maximize the visual impact of the colourful, fresh ingredients, serve this salad with the vegetables displayed in sections and the dressing in a bowl alongside ready to toss at the table.

serves 4   **prep** 10 mins   **cook** none

1 To make the dressing: whisk all the ingredients together. For a more emulsified finish, blend them in a small blender or food processor.

2 Spiralize the carrots, beetroot, cucumber, and squash. Divide the spiralized vegetables evenly among 4 bowls, laying out the vegetables in contrasting piles. Scatter each serving with the sesame seeds and coriander leaves. Serve with the dressing and lime halves alongside.

2 thick carrots, trimmed and peeled

1 medium beetroot, peeled

½ cucumber, trimmed

2 small summer squash or yellow heritage carrots, trimmed

1 tsp black sesame seeds, to garnish

coriander leaves, to garnish

lime halves, to serve

For the dressing

2 tbsp sunflower oil

2 tbsp lime juice

2 tsp sesame oil

2 tsp soy sauce

2 tsp honey

1 garlic clove, crushed

2.5cm (1in) piece fresh ginger root, peeled and finely grated

½ small shallot, finely chopped

Make it vegan

Replace the honey in the dressing with agave nectar or rice malt syrup.

Spicy Tahini Black Rice Noodle Salad

This stunning salad is tasty on its own as a light lunch or side dish, or topped with grilled teriyaki-glazed salmon as a main meal. Caramelized pumpkin seeds add a sweet and spicy crunch.

serves 4-6 **prep** 30 mins **cook** 5 mins

1 Preheat the oven to 180°C (350°F/Gas 4) and line a baking sheet with greaseproof paper. To make the caramelized pumpkin seeds: in a small bowl, whisk together the sunflower oil, sugar, salt, and chilli powder. Add the pumpkin seeds and toss to coat thoroughly, then spread on the prepared baking sheet. Bake on the top shelf of the oven for around 5 minutes, until the seeds begin to brown and stick together. Remove from the oven and spread on a plate to cool. Once cool, break up any clumps.

2 To make the dressing: whisk together all the ingredients along with 2 tablespoons cold water until completely combined. Set aside.

3 Cook the noodles according to the package instructions. Then drain, rinse well under cold water, and drain again. Toss with a drizzle of sunflower oil to prevent sticking. Allow to cool completely.

4 Use a potato peeler to peel wide ribbons of carrot into a serving bowl. Add the cabbage, spring onions, and most of the pumpkin seeds and coriander, along with the cooled noodles. Add the dressing and toss well to combine.

5 Heap the salad in the centre of the serving bowl. Sprinkle with the reserved pumpkin seeds and coriander. Season with salt and pepper to taste, and serve immediately.

300g (10oz) dried black rice noodles

sunflower oil, to toss

2 large carrots, peeled

200g (7oz) red cabbage, very finely sliced

4 spring onions, julienned

handful of coriander leaves, finely chopped

salt and freshly ground black pepper

For the pumpkin seeds

1 tsp sunflower oil

1 tbsp light brown sugar

pinch of salt

pinch of chilli powder

60g (2oz) raw shelled pumpkin seeds

For the dressing

2 tbsp tahini

2 tbsp sunflower oil

1 tsp chilli oil

2 tbsp lime juice

1 tbsp soy sauce

1 tbsp agave nectar

Make it with fish

For a main meal, top each salad with 100g (3½oz) grilled teriyaki-glazed salmon. Make the teriyaki glaze by combining 125ml (4½fl oz) each of water, mirin, soy sauce and sugar in a saucepan. Bring the mixture to a boil and stir until the sugar has dissolved. Simmer for 10–15 minutes or until the sauce thickens.

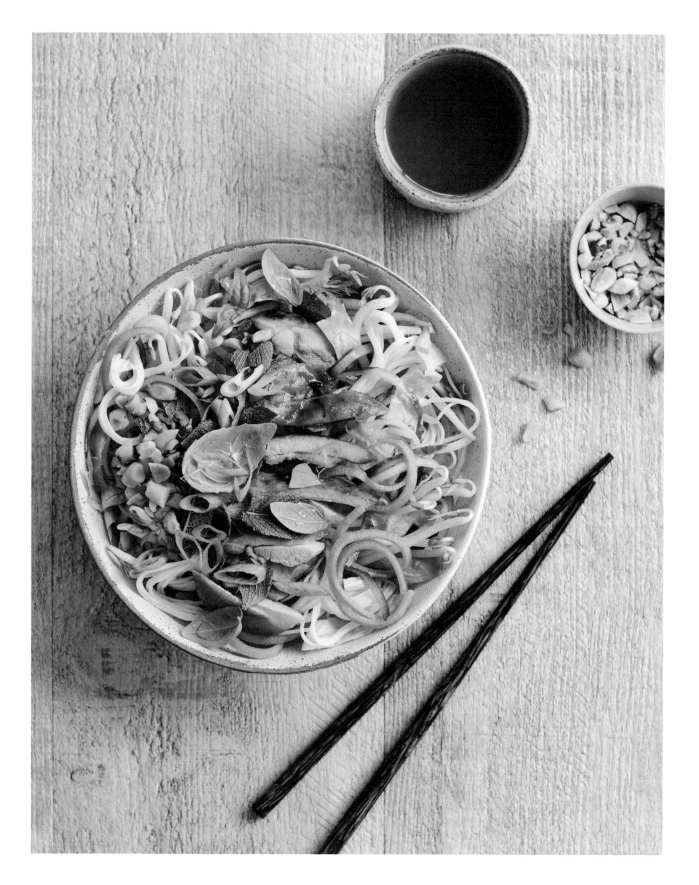

Vietnamese Chicken Noodle Salad

Based on the traditional Vietnamese dish of "bún", this refreshing noodle salad is tossed in a zesty citrus dressing and topped with chicken flavoured with ginger and lemongrass.

serves 4   **prep** 45 mins, plus marinating   **cook** 15 mins

1   To make the marinade: place all the ingredients in the bowl of a food processor and process until smooth.

2   With a rolling pin or meat mallet, pound the chicken thighs to flatten them to even thicknesses. Place in a shallow dish and add the marinade. Using your hands, rub the marinade into the chicken. Refrigerate, covered, for at least 2 hours and up to 12 hours.

3   To make the dressing: whisk together all the ingredients until the sugar has dissolved. Then whisk in 4 tablespoons cold water and set aside.

4   Place the noodles in a large, heatproof bowl and cover with boiling water. Leave to soak for 15 minutes until soft. Drain, rinse well under cold water, and drain again. Set aside to cool and drain completely.

5   Preheat the grill to high. Line a large, rimmed baking sheet with foil and arrange the marinated chicken in a single layer. Grill the chicken for 5 to 7 minutes on each side until dark brown and crispy in places. Set aside to cool slightly.

6   Divide the lettuce evenly among 4 bowls and top each bowl with an equal amount of noodles, spiralized cucumber and carrot, and bean sprouts. Lightly toss the ingredients in each bowl.

7   Top each bowl with 1 chicken thigh, sliced on the diagonal. Sprinkle with spring onions, mint, Thai basil, and peanuts. Serve immediately with the dressing on the side.

4 large skinless, boneless chicken thighs

300g (10oz) dried rice vermicelli

1 heart of cos lettuce, trimmed and shredded

¼ cucumber, spiralized

1 large, thick carrot, spiralized

2 large handfuls of bean sprouts

4 spring onions, finely sliced

handful of mint leaves, lightly chopped

handful of Thai basil, lightly chopped

2 heaped tbsp salted peanuts, roughly chopped

For the marinade

1 large or 2 small stalks lemongrass, peeled, trimmed, and finely chopped

1.5cm (½in) piece fresh ginger root, peeled and roughly chopped

1 garlic clove, roughly chopped

1 tbsp roughly chopped coriander stems

2 tbsp sunflower oil

1 tbsp lime juice

2 tsp light brown sugar

2 tsp soy sauce

2 tsp fish sauce

For the dressing

4 tbsp lemon juice

4 tsp fish sauce

3 tsp sugar

1 garlic clove, crushed

pinch of white pepper

Make it vegan

Replace the chicken with 450g (1lb) firm tofu cut into four pieces. Marinate the tofu according to step 2. Sear the pieces in a nonstick pan until they're golden brown and carmelised around the edges. Use extra soy sauce instead of fish sauce, too.

Mung Bean Gado Gado

Gado Gado is an Indonesian chopped salad whose name means "mix mix". It's always served with spicy peanut dressing, and is accompanied here by crisp vegetables and pulses.

serves 4   **prep** 45 mins   **cook** none

1 To make the spicy peanut dressing, in a small bowl whisk together the peanut butter, garlic powder, ginger, crushed dried chillies, soy sauce, lime juice, and vinegar. Stir in the water until thoroughly mixed. Set aside.

2 Adjust a spiralizer to the thinnest blade and spiralize the beetroot.

3 On a large serving plate, spread the cabbage in an even layer. On top of the cabbage, arrange in separate piles the cooked mung beans, cherry tomatoes, sprouted mung beans, spiralized beetroot, green beans, and hard-boiled eggs. Serve immediately with the dressing on the side.

125g (4½oz) smooth peanut butter

1 tsp garlic powder

1½ tsp ground ginger

1 tsp crushed dried chillies

1½ tsp soy sauce

juice of 2 limes

1 tsp rice wine vinegar

180ml (6fl oz) water

1 small beetroot, peeled

150g (5½oz) shredded Savoy cabbage

85g (3oz) cooked mung beans

85g (3oz) cherry tomatoes, halved

30g (1oz) sprouted mung beans (beansprouts)

75g (2½oz) green beans, chopped, blanched and drained

2 hard-boiled eggs, quartered

Why not try...

Use an equal amount of chickpeas in place of the cooked mung beans.

Make it vegan

Replace the eggs with 225g (8oz) diced and seared tempeh or tofu.

Make it with meat

Add to the serving plate a pile of 170g (6oz) thinly sliced, pan-seared steak.

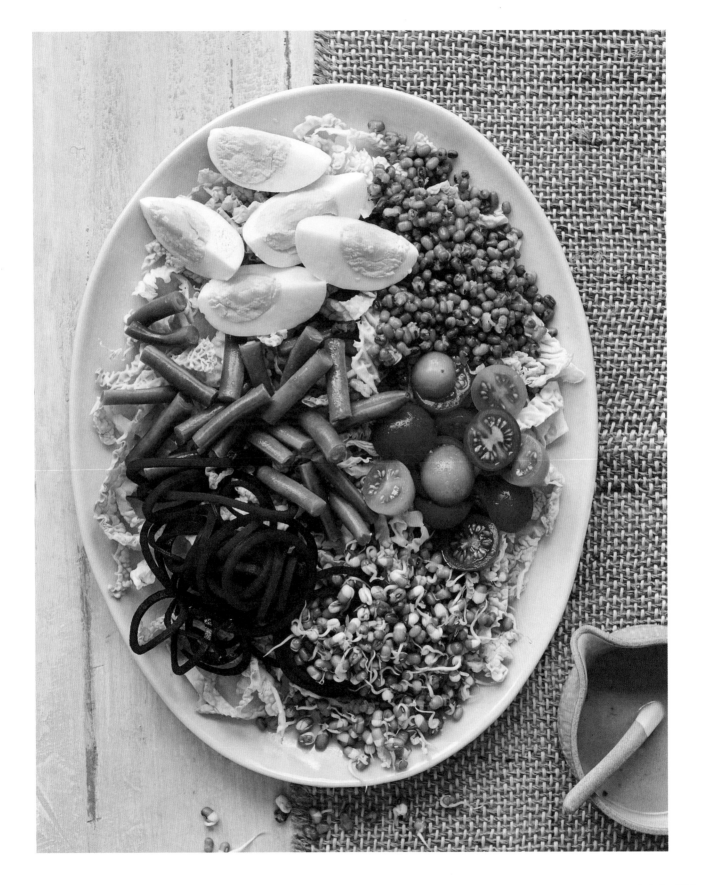

Roasted Carrots and Chickpeas

Vadouvan, or French masala, is a curry spice blend originating from Southern India. Cool yogurt tempers the spice and pairs well with the sweetness of roasted carrots.

serves 4   **prep** 15 mins   **cook** 30 mins

1   Preheat the oven to 150°C (350°F). Arrange the carrots in a single layer on a baking tray and drizzle with olive oil. Roast for 25–30 minutes until tender.

2   Meanwhile, in a small mixing bowl, toss together the chickpeas, vinegar, garlic, thyme, and crushed dried chillies. Season with salt and pepper. Set aside.

3   In another small mixing bowl, stir together the Greek-style yogurt and vadouvan.

4   Spread the yogurt on a serving plate, arrange the roasted carrots over the yogurt, and top with the chickpea mixture. Garnish with ground pepper and the reserved carrot leaves. Serve immediately.

450g (1lb) whole young carrots, leafy tops chopped and reserved for garnish

2 tbsp olive oil

350g (12oz) cooked chickpeas

2 tsp red wine vinegar

1 garlic clove, finely chopped

1 tsp thyme leaves

pinch of crushed dried chillies

salt and freshly ground black pepper

150g (5½oz) plain Greek-style yogurt

1 tbsp vadouvan (French masala)

Why not try...

If you can't find vadouvan, replace it with curry powder – it contains many of the same ingredients found in vadouvan.

Make it vegan

Substitute an equal amount of coconut yogurt (see page 38) for the Greek-style yogurt.

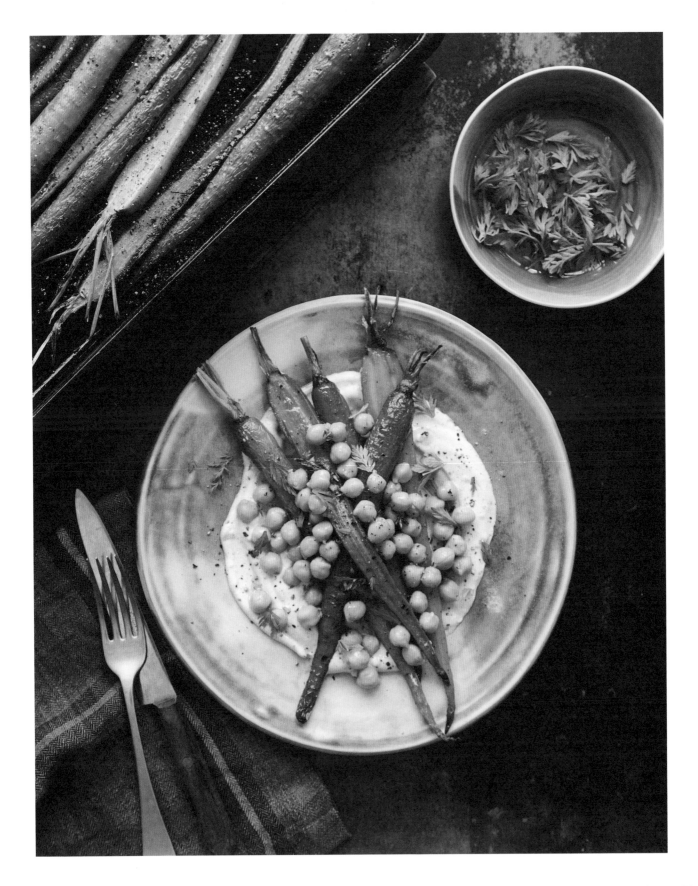

Avocado, Coriander, and Lime Tabbouleh

Tabbouleh is traditionally served as part of a mezze in the Middle East, but it also makes an excellent salad on its own or to accompany cold meats. The lime and avocado in this version give it a fresh dimension.

serves 4   **prep** 15 mins, plus soaking and chilling   **cook** none

1 Place 350ml (12fl oz) of water in a large saucepan and bring to the boil. Place the bulgur wheat and rock salt in a large bowl. Pour over the boiling water, cover, and leave to soak for about 30 minutes.

2 Drain any excess water from the bulgur wheat and place it in a large bowl. Then add the tomatoes, avocado, red peppers, onions, and coriander. Mix well to combine. Transfer the mixture to a large serving bowl.

3 Drizzle the lime juice and oil over the mixture. Toss well to coat. Season to taste with salt and black pepper, if needed. Mix well and chill the tabbouleh in the fridge for about 20 minutes before serving.

175g (6oz) bulgur wheat

1½ tsp rock salt

2 tomatoes, diced

1 avocado, peeled, pitted, and diced

1 small red pepper, deseeded and diced

60g (2oz) red onion, diced

handful of coriander leaves, roughly chopped

125ml (4¼fl oz) lime juice

2 tbsp extra virgin olive oil

salt and freshly ground black pepper

Make it with meat

This tabbouleh can be topped with grilled, sliced steak for a more filling meal.

Sweet Potato and Beluga Lentil Salad

The firm nuttiness of the lentils and the soft, caramelized sweet potato makes a wonderful combination of flavours and textures.

serves 2 **prep** 25 mins, plus cooling **cook** 45 mins

1. Preheat the oven to 180°C (350°F). On a baking tray, toss the sweet potato and paprika in 1 tablespoon of oil. Season with salt and pepper. Roast until tender and slightly caramelized, about 25 minutes, stirring once halfway. Let cool to room temperature.

2. Meanwhile, in a medium saucepan, bring the water to the boil. Add the lentils and return to the boil for 2–3 minutes. Reduce to a simmer and cook, covered, for 25–30 minutes, until tender but not soft. Drain in a fine colander and let cool to room temperature.

3. To assemble, in a large mixing bowl combine the lentils, sweet potatoes, onion, celery, and feta. Mix well. Drizzle in the honey, lemon juice, and remaining 1 tablespoon of oil. Toss to combine. Season with salt and pepper to taste. Garnish with the reserved celery leaves. Serve at room temperature.

1 large sweet potato, peeled and diced

⅛ tsp smoked paprika

2 tbsp olive oil

salt and freshly ground black pepper

750ml (1¼ pints) water

325g (11oz) uncooked beluga lentils

2 spring onions, trimmed and finely sliced

1 large celery stick, diced, leafy parts reserved for garnish

30g (1oz) feta cheese, crumbled

1 tbsp honey or agave nectar

juice of 1 lemon

Why not try...

Substitute an equal amount uncooked brown or green lentils for the beluga lentils.

Make it vegan

Use a nut-based vegan cheese alternative rather than feta.

Make it with meat

Add 4 crumbled rashers of crispy bacon to the lentil-feta mixture in step 3.

Butter Bean Panzanella

Panzanella is a Tuscan bread salad popular in the warmer months. It's a great use for day-old bread and wonderful for parties and picnics, as it can be served at room temperature.

serves 6   **prep** 25 mins   **cook** 15 mins

1 Preheat the oven to 170°C (325°F). Cut the bread into 1cm (½in) cubes. On a baking sheet, arrange the bread cubes in a single layer and bake for 15 minutes, or until toasted and light golden brown.

2 Meanwhile, to make the dressing, in a small bowl whisk together the vinegar and Dijon mustard. While whisking, drizzle in the oil and thoroughly combine. Stir in the garlic, oregano, and basil. Set aside.

3 To assemble, in a large salad bowl, add the tomatoes, butter beans, cucumber, and sweetcorn. Fold in the toasted bread, then drizzle the dressing over. Toss to coat. Season with salt and pepper to taste. Serve immediately.

1 small loaf sourdough bread

60ml (2fl oz) red wine vinegar

1 tbsp Dijon mustard

120ml (4fl oz) olive oil

2 garlic cloves, finely chopped

1 tsp chopped oregano

1 tsp chopped basil leaves

175g (6oz) cherry tomatoes, halved

225g (8oz) cooked butter beans

1 cucumber, diced

150g (5½oz) fresh sweetcorn kernels

salt and freshly ground
   black pepper

Make it with fish

Add 115g (4oz) cooked prawns when you assemble the salad.

Caprese Farro Salad

Featuring fresh summer tomatoes, soft mozzarella, chewy farro, and a homemade pesto sauce, this colourful and light Italian salad makes the perfect starter for any meal.

serves 4   **prep** 10 mins, plus cooling   **cook** 50 mins

1 Rinse the farro under cold running water and place in a large saucepan. Cover with about 600ml (1 pint) of water and bring to the boil. Then reduce the heat to a simmer and cook, stirring occasionally, for about 40 minutes or until softened. Remove from the heat, drain, and set aside to cool.

2 For the pesto, place the basil leaves, pine nuts, garlic, and oil in a food processor and pulse until smooth. Season to taste, if needed.

3 Place the mozzarella and tomatoes in a large bowl. Add the pesto and cooled farro and stir to mix. Chill the salad in the fridge until ready to serve, garnished with a few basil leaves.

200g (7oz) uncooked farro

225g (8oz) mozzarella cheese, diced

3 large tomatoes, cut into bite-sized pieces

For the pesto

45g (1½oz) basil leaves, rinsed and dried, plus extra to garnish

2 tbsp pine nuts

1 garlic clove

2–3 tbsp extra virgin olive oil

salt

Why not try...

You could replace the fresh mozzarella cheese with the same quantity of burrata cheese.

Make it vegan

Use a nut cheese (see page 37) instead of the mozzarella.

Nutty Barley and Lentil Salad

This is no boring salad! The combination of hearty barley and nutty, crunchy almonds and walnuts is well balanced by the contrasting tastes and textures of sweet, dried cranberries and salty goat's cheese.

serves 4   **prep** 10 mins, plus overnight soaking and cooling   **cook** 30 mins

1 Place the barley in a bowl, cover with water, and leave to soak overnight or for at least 8 hours. Then drain, rinse under running water, and drain well again.

2 Place the barley in a lidded saucepan and cover with plenty of water. Bring to the boil, then reduce the heat to a simmer, and cover. Cook for about 30 minutes or until the barley is tender. Remove from the heat, drain any remaining water, and leave to cool completely.

3 Once cooled, place the barley and lentils in a large bowl and mix lightly to combine. Add the almonds, walnuts, and cranberries and mix to combine. Sprinkle over the goat's cheese, add the rocket, and toss lightly. Divide the salad equally between four plates and serve immediately.

75g (2½oz) uncooked pearl barley

400g can green lentils, drained

25g (scant 1oz) almonds, roughly chopped

25g (scant 1oz) walnuts, roughly chopped

50g (1¾oz) dried cranberries

100g (3½oz) soft goat's cheese, crumbled

100g (3½oz) rocket

Why not try...

You could try the same amount of sunflower seeds or chopped Brazil nuts instead of the almonds or walnuts. You could also replace the rocket with the same quantity of flat-leaf parsley.

Make it vegan

Simply replace the soft goat's cheese with nut cheese (see page 37).

Freekeh Sweet and Spicy Warm Salad

This warming and colourful salad combines sweet roasted squash and sticky dates with a fragrant and spiced freekeh and is perfect for autumn and winter lunches.

serves 4 **prep** 15 mins, plus cooling **cook** 40 mins

1 Preheat the oven to 200°C (400°F/Gas 6). Place the cinnamon, ginger, cumin, and oil in a small bowl and mix to combine. Place the butternut squash in a baking tray, pour the mixture over, and toss to coat. Bake in the oven for 30–35 minutes or until the squash is tender.

2 Meanwhile, rinse the freekeh under running water and place in a large saucepan. Cover with 1 litre (1¾ pints) of water and bring to the boil. Then reduce the heat to a simmer and cook for 15 minutes or until almost all the water has been absorbed. Remove from the heat, drain any remaining water, and leave to cool slightly.

3 For the dressing, place all the ingredients in a bowl. Season to taste and mix to combine. Place the radicchio and dates in a large serving dish. Add the squash and freekeh and toss lightly to mix. Then pour over the dressing, season to taste, and toss until well combined. Serve warm garnished with parsley.

2 tsp ground cinnamon

1 tsp grated ginger

1 tsp ground cumin

2 tbsp light olive oil

1 butternut squash, deseeded and cut into 2cm (¾in) cubes

200g (7oz) cracked freekeh

1 small head radicchio, roughly chopped

8 dried pitted dates, about 40g (1½oz) in total, roughly chopped

4 tbsp roughly chopped flat-leaf parsley

For the dressing

4 tbsp extra virgin olive oil

juice of 1 lemon

1 tbsp honey

salt and freshly ground black pepper

Why not try...

Try using 2 large sweet potatoes in place of the squash, and cook in the same way. You can also use chicory or rocket leaves instead of the radicchio.

Make it vegan

Use maple syrup or agave nectar instead of honey.

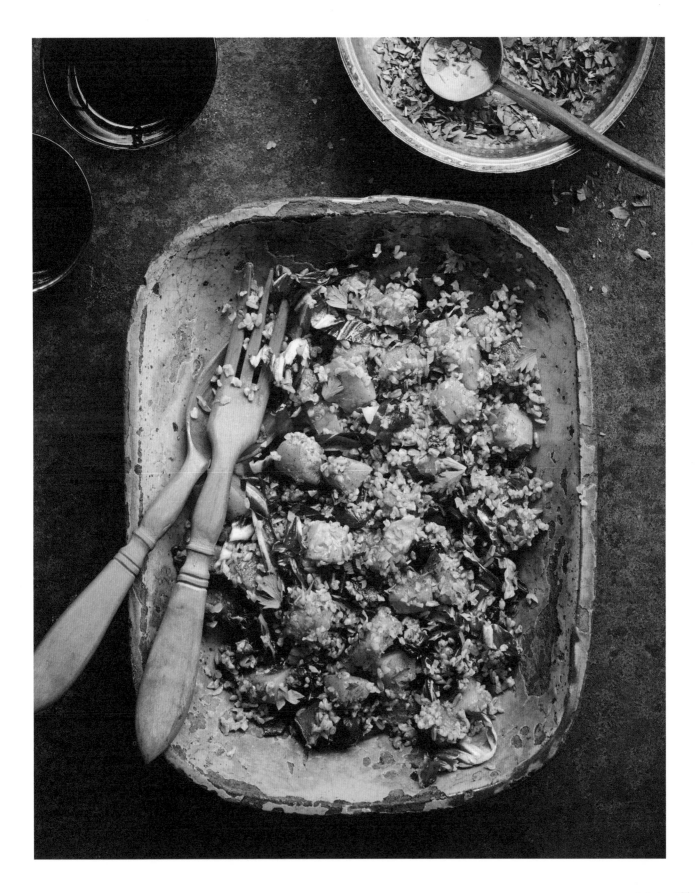

Soups and Stews

From ramen and minestrone to chilli, the variety of soups and stews in this chapter are perfect for expanding your cooking repertoire and impressing dinner guests. Get into the habit of making double batches to store in the freezer, ensuring you'll always have delicious, nutritious meals on hand.

Mushroom Miso Ramen

A light, miso-based soup, this ramen will appeal to mushroom lovers, as it contains three different types. The mushrooms bring an earthy flavour to the ramen, which pairs very well with both the tofu and miso.

serves 4   **prep** 10 mins   **cook** 30 mins

1   In a large pan over a medium heat, bring the stock to a simmer.

2   Add the oyster mushrooms, shiitake mushrooms, and spring onions, and simmer for 20 minutes.

3   Add the vegetarian white miso paste, tofu, and baby spinach. Simmer for 5 minutes.

4   While the broth is simmering, in a large pan of boiling water over a high heat, cook the ramen noodles for 4 minutes, stirring occasionally. Drain, rinse, and divide between 4 deep serving bowls.

5   Fill the bowls with the hot broth, just covering the noodles.

6   Add the enoki mushrooms and nori strips to each bowl, then serve.

1.4 litres (2½ pints) Vegan Ramen Stock (see page 31)

85g (3oz) oyster mushrooms, sliced

85g (3oz) shiitake mushrooms

8 spring onions, finely chopped (reserve some green for garnish)

4 tbsp vegetarian white miso paste

175g (6oz) firm tofu, diced

85g (3oz) baby spinach

680g (24oz) ramen noodles

175g (6oz) fresh enoki mushrooms, trimmed

4 sheets nori, sliced into strips

Tom Yum Ramen

Tom Yum hails from Thailand. With its light, creamy texture and citrusy flavour, this dish is balanced and refreshing. You can serve this ramen on a hot summer night with a crisp, cool drink.

serves 4   **prep** 25 mins   **cook** 40 mins

1 In a large pan over a medium heat, bring the stock to a simmer.

2 Add the garlic, galangal, lemongrass, and makrut lime leaves. Cover the pan, and simmer for 30 minutes. Strain the broth, discarding the solids.

3 Bring the broth back up to a simmer and add the Thai chilli garlic paste, salt, sugar, white soy sauce, lime juice (to taste), oyster mushrooms, cherry tomatoes, tofu, and coconut milk. Simmer for 5 minutes.

4 While the broth is simmering, in a large pan of boiling water over a high heat, cook the ramen noodles for 4 minutes, stirring occasionally. Drain, rinse, and divide between 4 deep serving bowls.

5 Fill the bowls with the hot broth, just covering the noodles. Garnish each bowl with the spring onions and coriander, and serve with the lime wedges.

1.4 litres (2½ pints) Vegan Ramen Stock (see page 31)

4 garlic cloves, finely chopped

5cm (2in) knob galangal or ginger, sliced

2 whole stalks lemongrass, peeled and chopped in 7.5cm (3in) pieces

3 makrut (kaffir) lime leaves

2 tsp Thai chilli garlic paste

1 tsp sea salt

1½ tsp sugar

2 tbsp white soy sauce

juice of 1 lime

175g (6oz) oyster mushrooms, trimmed

8 cherry tomatoes

175g (6oz) firm tofu, diced

120ml (4fl oz) coconut milk

680g (24oz) ramen noodles

45g (1½oz) spring onions, finely chopped

45g (1½oz) coriander, roughly chopped

1 lime, cut into 4 wedges

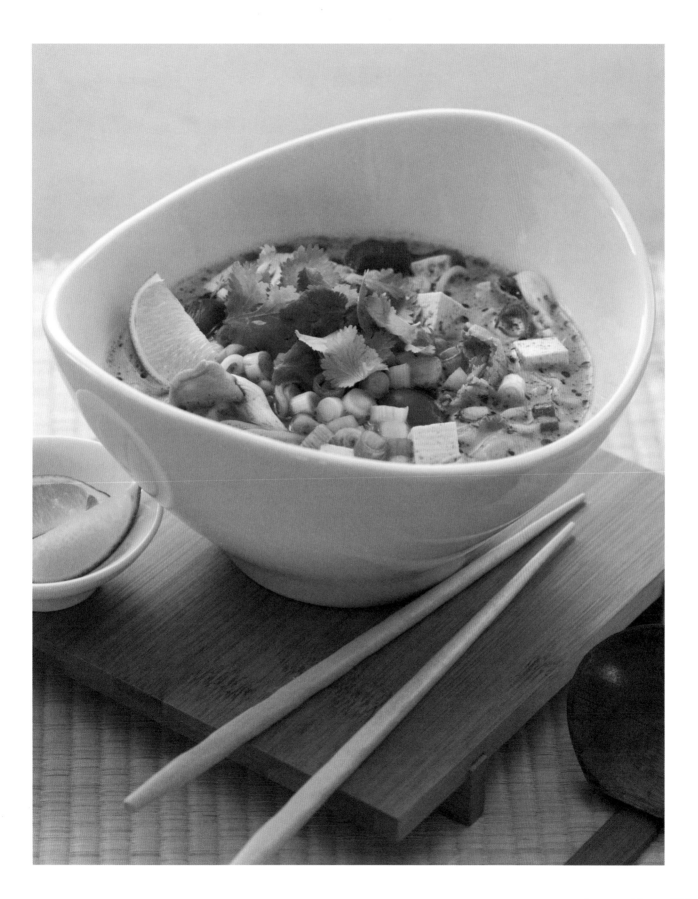

Tomato Miso Ramen

This ramen is as comforting as a bowl of tomato soup, but with the added depth of salty miso and the addition of delicious, chewy noodles.

serves 4　**prep** 20 mins　**cook** 15 mins

1　In a large pan over a medium heat, bring the stock to a simmer.

2　Chop the tomatoes into bite-sized pieces, and add to the broth.

3　Add the tomato purée, sugar, and white soy sauce. Simmer for 5 minutes.

4　Add the vegetarian red miso paste and chilli bean paste. Simmer for 5 minutes.

5　While the broth is simmering, in a large pan of boiling water over a high heat, cook the ramen noodles for 4 minutes, stirring occasionally. Drain, rinse, and divide between 4 deep serving bowls.

6　Fill the bowls with the hot broth, just covering the noodles.

7　Garnish each bowl with the spring onions, and serve with lime wedges.

1.4 litres (2½ pints) Vegan Ramen Stock (see page 31)

6 tomatoes, cored and peeled

1 tbsp tomato purée

1 tbsp sugar

1 tbsp white soy sauce

3 tbsp vegetarian red miso paste

2 tsp fermented chilli bean paste

680g (24oz) ramen noodles

45g (1½oz) spring onions, finely chopped

1 lime, cut into 4 wedges

Coconut Curry Tofu Ramen

Coconut milk and curry powder are a wonderful marriage of creamy and sharp flavours. Lime juice is an important addition that highlights and balances the curry. Coriander finishes this dish with a bold, fresh flavour.

serves 4   **prep** 20 mins   **cook** 15 mins

1   In a large pan over a medium heat, bring the stock to a simmer.

2   Add the coconut milk, ginger, salt, curry powder, button mushrooms, crushed chilli flakes, mirin, white soy sauce, and sugar. Simmer for 5 minutes.

3   Add the tofu, baby spinach, and lime juice. Simmer for 5 minutes.

4   While the broth is simmering, in a large pan of boiling water over a high heat, cook the ramen noodles for 4 minutes, stirring occasionally. Drain, rinse, and divide between 4 deep serving bowls.

5   Fill the serving bowls with the hot broth, just covering the noodles.

6   Garnish each bowl with the soft-boiled eggs, spring onions, and coriander.

1.4 litres (2½ pints) Vegan Ramen Stock (see page 31)

120ml (4fl oz) coconut milk

1 tsp grated ginger

1 tsp sea salt

2 tsp curry powder

8 button mushrooms, thinly sliced

1 tsp crushed chilli flakes

2½ tbsp mirin

1 tbsp white soy sauce

1 tsp sugar

175g (6oz) tofu, diced

85g (3oz) baby spinach

1½ tbsp lime juice

680g (24oz) ramen noodles

4 soft-boiled eggs, sliced in half lengthways

45g (1½oz) spring onions, finely chopped

45g (1½oz) coriander, roughly chopped

Make it vegan

Instead of the hard-boiled eggs, top the ramen with another vegetable, such as miso-glazed roasted aubergine.

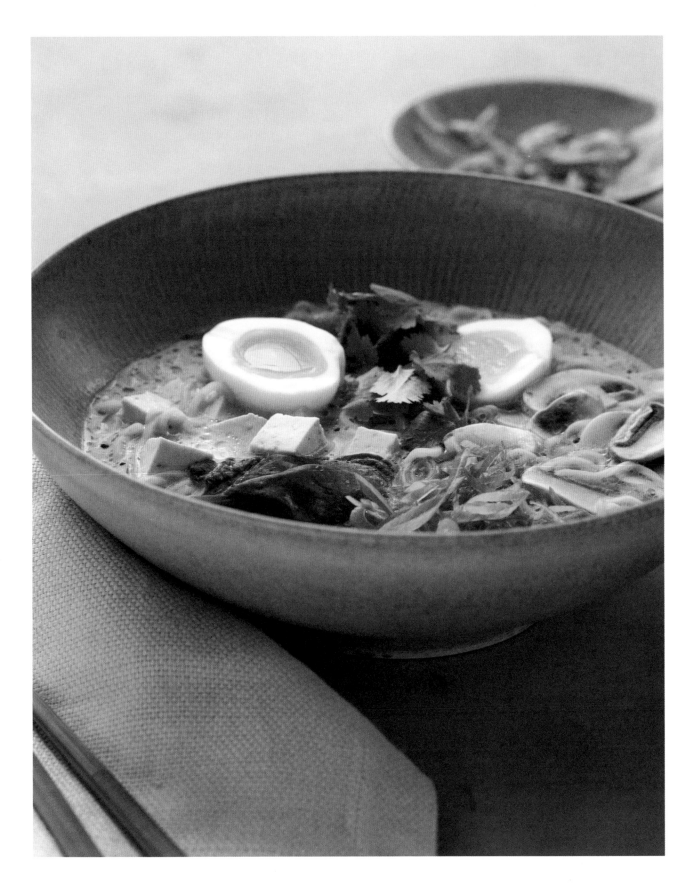

Sweetcorn Chowder Ramen

Fresh sweetcorn is the star of this vegetarian ramen dish. It's enhanced by the salty, complex flavour of the miso. The addition of cream provides a lovely richness to the ramen.

serves 4   **prep** 20 mins   **cook** 15 mins

1 Heat the vegetable oil in a large pan over a medium heat. Add the onion, and sauté until translucent. Add the garlic, and sauté for 1 minute, until fragrant.

2 Add the stock, 350g (12oz) sweetcorn, cream, vegetarian white miso paste, mirin, and salt. Simmer for 10 minutes.

3 Using a hand-held blender, blend the broth until much of the sweetcorn has been incorporated, while still leaving some larger kernel chunks. Add the remaining sweetcorn, and simmer for 5 minutes.

4 While the broth is simmering, in a large pan of boiling water over a high heat, cook the ramen noodles for 50 seconds, stirring occasionally. Drain, rinse, and divide between 4 deep serving bowls.

5 Fill the bowls with the hot broth, just covering the noodles. Place 1 knob butter in the middle of each bowl, and sprinkle with the chives.

1 tbsp vegetable oil

1 litre (1¾ pints) Vegan Ramen Stock (see page 31)

1 small onion, diced

1 clove garlic, finely chopped

500g (1lb 2oz) cooked sweetcorn kernels

500ml (16fl oz) single cream

2½ tbsp vegetarian white miso paste

2 tsp mirin

1 tsp sea salt

680g (24oz) fresh ramen noodles

4 knobs butter (about 2 tbsp)

50g (1¾oz) chives, finely chopped

Make it with meat

Add 85g (3oz) cooked, sliced chicken breast atop each bowl.

Soups and Stews **147**

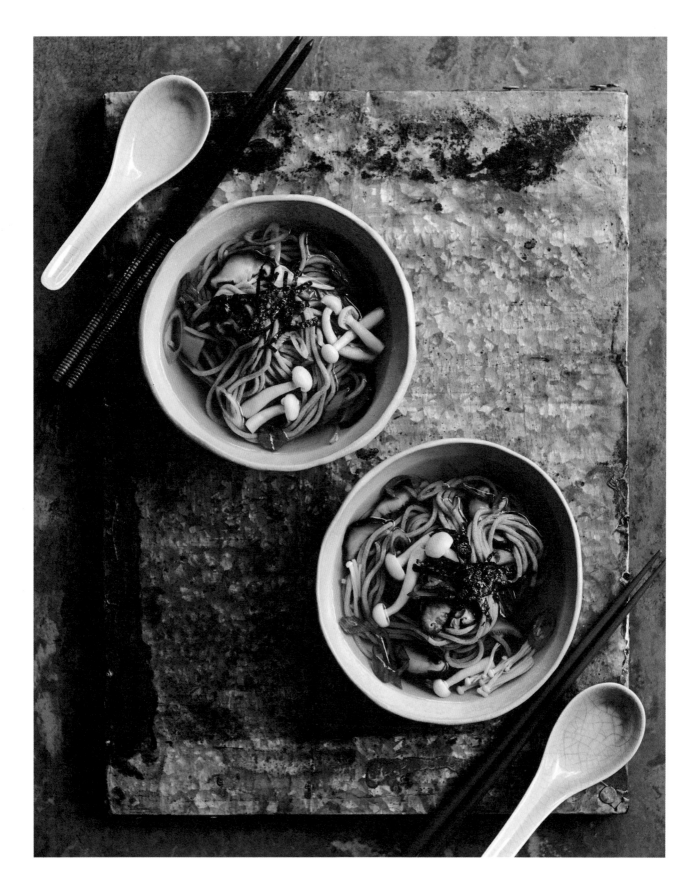

Buckwheat Noodle Soup with Enoki and Shiitake

Making your own dashi, or Japanese stock, is a very simple affair that creates a delicate yet flavoursome soup base. Here both dried and fresh shiitake are used to make a vegetarian version.

serves 4 **prep** 20 mins, plus soaking **cook** 15 mins

1 To make the dashi: place the dried kombu, dried shiitake mushrooms, and fresh shiitake mushroom stalks in a saucepan and cover with 1.2 litres (2 pints) cold water. Soak for 1 to 3 hours.

2 After soaking, bring the dashi almost to the boil over a medium heat, but remove from the heat just before it boils. Season with salt, and stir in the rice vinegar and soy sauce. Remove and discard the kombu, and let the dashi cool. Strain the dashi through a sieve lined with kitchen paper to remove the shiitake mushrooms.

3 Cook the noodles in boiling, salted water for 3 to 4 minutes until just al dente. Drain and rinse well under cold water.

4 In a large saucepan, bring the dashi to the boil over a medium-high heat. Add the enoki mushrooms, spring onions, shiitake mushroom caps, and noodles. Return to the boil until the noodles are heated through and the mushrooms are soft. Remove from the heat and season to taste with salt. Serve immediately, topped with seaweed strips.

300g buckwheat soba noodles

60g (2oz) fresh enoki mushrooms

4 spring onions, finely sliced on the diagonal

8 small seaweed snack sheets (kim nori), cut into thin strips, to garnish

For the dashi

15g (½oz) dried kombu, cut into pieces

15g (½oz) dried shiitake mushrooms

60g (2oz) fresh shiitake mushrooms, stalks and caps separate, and caps thinly sliced

salt

1 tsp rice vinegar

1 tbsp soy sauce

Thai Curry, Tomato and Vegetable Soup with Farro

Tomato soup takes on a whole new life in this recipe, when mixed with Thai curry paste and a variety of fresh vegetables. The addition of farro gives just the right amount of bulk to this satisfying soup.

serves 4   **prep** 10 mins   **cook** 1 hr 30 mins

1 Place the farro in a large, lidded saucepan and cover with water. Place over a medium heat, cover, and simmer for about 1 hour or until almost all the water has been absorbed. Drain any remaining water and set aside.

2 Place a large, lidded saucepan over a medium heat. Add the coconut milk, stock, tomato purée, Thai red curry paste, and sugar and stir to combine. Cover and bring to the boil, stirring occasionally to make sure the ingredients are well combined. Then reduce the heat to a low simmer and cook the soup for a further 20 minutes.

3 Meanwhile, heat the oil in a large frying pan over a medium heat. Add the leeks and green peppers and sauté for 10 minutes or until softened and browned in places. Add the courgette and cook for a further 3 minutes. Remove from the heat and set aside.

4 Add the tomatoes to the soup. Taste and adjust the seasoning and cook the soup, stirring once, for 5 minutes. Then add the leek mixture and the farro. Stir well to mix and remove from the heat. Ladle the soup into bowls and garnish with coriander. Serve hot with a green salad and crusty ciabatta bread.

75g (2½oz) uncooked farro

400g can light coconut milk

200ml (7fl oz) vegetable stock

175g (6oz) tomato purée

2 tbsp Thai red curry paste

1 tbsp light brown sugar

1 tbsp extra virgin olive oil

2 leeks, white and light green parts only, chopped

1 green pepper, deseeded and diced

1 courgette, diced

1 large beef tomato, diced

sea salt and freshly ground black pepper

handful of coriander leaves, to garnish

Make it with fish

Marinate 4 snapper fillets or other firm white fish in 2 tbsp lime juice and 2 tsp sea salt for 30 minutes. Add the fish to the soup in step 4 and gently simmer for 6 to 8 minutes, or until the fish is just cooked through.

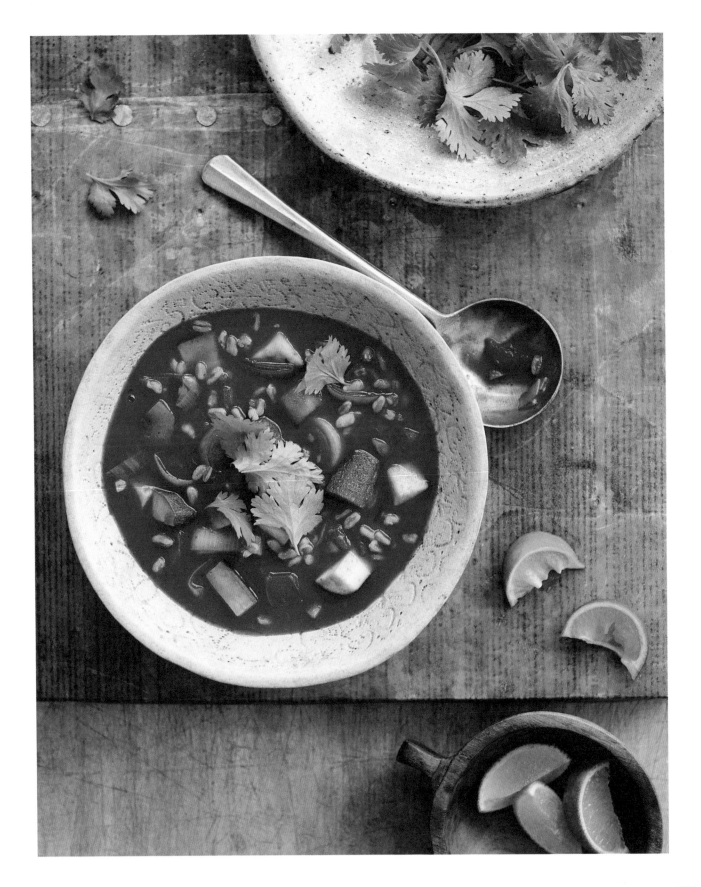

Green Minestrone with Kale and Walnut Pesto

This bright, vibrant soup is made with a variety of fresh spring vegetables that give it a tender-crisp texture. Be sure to add them to the soup in the correct order, so they are all cooked al dente.

serves 4-6 **prep** 35 mins **cook** 15 mins

1 To make the pesto: in a large, non-stick frying pan, dry-fry the walnuts over a medium–low heat for 3 to 4 minutes, stirring frequently, until they start to brown. Remove from the heat. Once cool, rub them well in a clean tea towel to remove the skins. Roughly chop.

2 In a food processor, pulse the walnuts, kale, garlic, lemon juice, basil, olive oil, and 2 tablespoons cold water to form a rough paste. Add the Parmesan and pulse until you reach the desired consistency, adding a little extra olive oil if necessary. The pesto should not be completely smooth. Taste and season with salt and pepper, and pulse once more to combine.

3 Cook the pasta according to the package instructions. Drain and rinse the cooked pasta under cold water. Toss with a drizzle of olive oil to prevent sticking. Set aside.

4 In a large, heavy-based saucepan, heat the olive oil over a medium heat. Add the onion, celery, and fennel, and cook for 3 to 4 minutes, stirring occasionally, until soft but not brown. Then add the garlic and cook for 1 minute more.

5 Add the vegetable stock and bring to the boil. Add the green beans and cook for 1 minute. Add the asparagus and peas and cook for 2 minutes more. Finally, add the courgette and pasta and cook for a final minute. Taste and season with salt and pepper. Serve immediately, with pesto alongside for topping.

115g (4oz) pasta tubes or orzo

2 tbsp olive oil, plus extra to toss

1 small yellow onion, finely diced

1 celery stalk, finely diced

⅓ large fennel bulb, finely diced

1 large garlic clove, finely chopped

1.4 litres (2½ pints) vegetable stock

large handful of young green beans, finely sliced

10 asparagus spears, finely sliced

60g (2oz) frozen peas

½ small courgette, halved lengthways and finely sliced

For the pesto

60g (2oz) walnut halves

30g (1oz) young kale, washed, de-veined, and shredded

1 large garlic clove, crushed

2 tbsp lemon juice

12 basil leaves

4 tbsp olive oil

2 tbsp grated Parmesan cheese

salt and freshly ground black pepper

Make it vegan

Use a plant-based Parmesan cheese or nutritional yeast instead of Parmesan cheese, and ensure the pasta is eggless.

Creamy Spinach and Mung Bean Soup

Don't let the bright colour fool you – this soup is as luxurious as it is good for you, and especially tasty with freshly baked bread.

serves 4   **prep** 25 mins   **cook** 40 mins

1 In a flameproof casserole or stock pot, melt the butter over a medium heat. Add the onion and cook for 3-4 minutes until translucent. Add the garlic and cook for 2 minutes.

2 Add the potato and stir to combine. Cook for 2-3 minutes. Add 500ml (16fl oz) stock and bring to the boil. Reduce the heat to a simmer and cook, covered, for 12-15 minutes, until the potatoes are tender.

3 Add the spinach and mung beans and cook for an additional 5 minutes, or until the spinach wilts and the mung beans are warmed through. Leave to cool.

4 With a blender (working in batches) or a hand-held blender, purée the soup until smooth. Return the puréed mixture to the pan and stir in the sherry, cayenne, and nutmeg. For a thinner consistency, add some of the remaining stock as desired. Season with salt and pepper to taste.

5 Reheat the soup over a medium heat. Transfer to serving bowls and top with Parmesan. Serve immediately.

1 tbsp unsalted butter

1 onion, diced

1 garlic clove, finely chopped

1 potato, peeled and cut into 1cm (½in) chunks

750ml (1¼ pints) vegetable stock

175g (6oz) baby spinach

175g (6oz) cooked mung beans

2 tbsp dry sherry

⅛ tsp ground cayenne pepper

⅛ tsp ground nutmeg

salt and freshly ground black pepper

20g (¾oz) grated Parmesan cheese

Why not try...

Garnish with flat-leaf parsley or watercress for a more pronounced green flavour.

Make it vegan

Replace the butter with an equal amount of coconut oil, and use a plant-based Parmesan cheese.

Make it with meat

Crumble 1 tbsp crisped prosciutto on top of each bowl of soup.

Pigeon Pea and Pumpkin Chilli

Pumpkin may seem like an unusual ingredient in chilli, but its sweetness is a lovely complement to the spiciness of this soup.

serves 6 **prep** 25 mins **cook** 45 mins

1 In a large stock pot, heat the oil over a medium-low heat. Add the onion and cook for 2–3 minutes until soft. Add the garlic and jalapeño and cook for an additional minute.

2 Incorporate the tomatoes, cumin, and chipotle chilli powder. Stir in the stock, bring to the boil, reduce the heat and then simmer for 5 minutes. Stir in the pigeon peas (or black-eyed beans), adzuki beans, and sweetcorn. Return to the boil then reduce the heat to low and simmer, covered, for 20 minutes.

3 Fold in the pumpkin and stir to combine. Cook, covered, for another 10 minutes. Season with salt and pepper to taste. Transfer to 6 serving bowls, garnish with the chopped coriander, and serve immediately.

1 tbsp olive oil

1 small onion, diced

2 garlic cloves, finely chopped

1 small jalapeño, deseeded and minced

400g can chopped tomatoes

2½ tsp ground cumin

1½ tsp chipotle chilli powder

500ml (16fl oz) vegetable stock

375g (13oz) cooked pigeon peas or black-eyed beans

400g (14oz) cooked adzuki beans

115g (4oz) sweetcorn kernels

425g can pure pumpkin

salt and freshly ground black pepper

60g (2oz) chopped coriander leaves, to garnish

Make it with meat

Cook 225g (8oz) raw turkey mince along with the onion in step 1.

Chickpea and Haricot Bean Bisque

While not a traditional bisque, this soup certainly seems like one with its silky, rich texture. This simple, elegant recipe makes an excellent first course for a dinner party.

serves 4   **prep** 15 mins   **cook** 30 mins

1 In a flameproof casserole or large saucepan, warm the oil over a medium-low heat until shimmering. Add the leek and cook for 4–5 minutes until soft and translucent. Add the garlic and cook for an additional 2 minutes.

2 Add the vermouth and cook for 1–2 minutes. Incorporate the stock, haricot beans, and chickpeas. Bring to the boil, then reduce to a simmer and cook, covered, for 15 minutes. Remove from the heat and leave to cool for 5–10 minutes.

3 Transfer the mixture to a blender and purée until smooth. Return to the pan over a medium heat, stir in the cream, and heat. Season with salt and pepper to taste. Transfer to serving bowls, garnish with the hazelnuts and a swirl of oil, and serve immediately.

½ tbsp olive oil, plus extra to garnish

1 leek, white parts only, sliced

1 garlic clove, finely chopped

1 tbsp dry vermouth

750ml (1¼ pints) vegetable stock

450g (1lb) cooked haricot beans

175g (6oz) cooked chickpeas

60ml (2fl oz) double cream

salt and freshly ground black pepper

chopped toasted hazelnuts, to garnish

Make it vegan

The cooked chickpeas are naturally creamy, so you can easily omit the double cream for a vegan-friendly version

Brazilian Black Bean and Pumpkin Stew

A colourful and gutsy dish, you could always add some spicy sausage or chorizo if you prefer a meaty meal. Black beans are also called turtle beans and need soaking overnight.

serves 4-6   **prep** 25 mins, plus soaking   **cook** 2½-3 hrs

1 Preheat the oven to 160°C (325°F/Gas 3). Put the beans in a large heavy-based pan and cover with water. Bring to the boil, then reduce to a simmer, partially cover with the lid, and cook on a low heat for 1 hour. Drain and set aside.

2 Heat the oil in a large heavy-based pan over a medium heat, add the onion, and cook for 3-4 minutes until soft. Season with salt and pepper, stir in the garlic, and cook for 1-2 minutes until soft. Stir in the pumpkin or butternut squash, red peppers, tomatoes, and chilli.

3 Add the beans, pour over the stock, and bring to the boil. Then reduce to a simmer, cover with the lid and put in the oven for 1½-2 hours. Taste and season, if necessary, then stir through the mango and coriander. Serve with some soured cream and rice on the side.

325g (11oz) dried black beans, soaked overnight and drained

1 tbsp olive oil

1 onion, finely chopped

salt and freshly ground black pepper

3 garlic cloves, finely chopped

1 small pumpkin or butternut squash, peeled, deseeded, and diced

2 red peppers, deseeded and diced

2 × 400g cans chopped tomatoes

1 small green chilli, deseeded and diced

900ml (1½ pint) hot vegetable stock

1 mango, peeled, stone removed, and diced

bunch of coriander, chopped

Make it with meat

Add 250g (9oz) chopped spicy sausage or chorizo to the pan in step 2 after adding the garlic. Cook for 6-8 minutes until seared.

Kitchari Stew with Kamut

The word "kitchari" literally means mixture, and is an Indian recipe that mixes two or more grains for a soothing and warming dish. This recipe uses kamut instead of rice, for more texture and bite.

serves 3 **prep** 10 mins, plus overnight soaking **cook** 2 hrs 10 mins

1 Place the peas in a large bowl, cover with water, and leave to soak for about 12 hours. Place the kamut in a separate bowl, cover with water, and leave to soak overnight or for up to 8 hours. Drain any remaining water from the peas and kamut. Rinse under running water, drain well, and set aside.

2 Heat the oil in a large, lidded saucepan over a medium heat. Add the ginger, turmeric, cumin, coriander, and cinnamon. Reduce the heat to low and cook for 1–2 minutes, stirring frequently, making sure the spices do not burn.

3 Add the peas, kamut, and 1.5 litres (2¾ pints) of water to the pan. Season with salt and bring the mixture to a simmer. Cover partially and cook, stirring occasionally, for 2 hours or until the peas have broken down and the kamut is tender and chewy. Taste and adjust the seasoning, if needed. Remove from the heat and garnish with coriander. Serve hot.

150g (5½oz) yellow split peas

100g (3½oz) uncooked kamut

1 tbsp coconut oil or ghee

5cm (2in) piece of fresh root ginger, finely chopped

2 tsp turmeric

2 tsp ground cumin

1 tsp ground coriander

½ tsp ground cinnamon

salt

handful of coriander leaves, to garnish

Why not try...

If you can't find kamut, stick with the traditional version of this dish and use basmati rice. Add 100g (3½oz) rinsed basmati rice with the soaked peas and water in step 3. You should only need to simmer for 1 hour, stirring periodically as the rice may stick to the bottom of the pan.

Red Wine-Braised Beetroot and Lentils with Farro

Beetroot and lentils are a match made in heaven when braised in a full-bodied red wine. Be sure to use a wine of good quality, as it will enhance the flavour of the stew and you can save a glass to have with your meal.

serves 4   **prep** 30 mins, plus overnight soaking and chilling   **cook** 1 hr 20 mins

1   Place the farro in a large bowl, cover with water, and leave to soak overnight or for up to 12 hours. Then drain and rinse under running water. Drain well.

2   Heat 1 tablespoon of the light olive oil in a saucepan over a medium heat. Add the farro and sliced garlic. Season to taste with salt and cook for 5 minutes, stirring occasionally, until the farro is lightly toasted. Add 900ml (1½ pints) of water and bring to the boil. Then reduce the heat to a simmer, cover, and cook for 25–30 minutes or until the farro is tender. Drain any remaining water and rinse under running water. Drain well and set aside.

3   For the lentils and vegetables, heat the remaining light olive oil in a large, heavy-based, lidded saucepan over a medium heat. Add the onions and cook for 2–3 minutes or until softened. Then add the garlic, beetroot, and carrots. Season to taste with a good grinding of pepper and cook for 5–10 minutes, stirring occasionally. Add the tomato purée in a corner of the pan, cook for 1–2 minutes, then stir to mix with the vegetables.

4   Add the lentils, wine, stock, rosemary, thyme, and bay leaf. Bring to the boil. Then reduce the heat to a simmer and cook, covered, for 25 minutes or until the lentils and vegetables are cooked through. Season with salt and cook for a further 5–10 minutes. Remove from the heat and discard the rosemary, thyme, and bay leaf.

5   Place the yogurt, lemon juice, lemon zest, crushed garlic, and extra virgin olive oil in a bowl. Finely chop the parsley and add to the bowl. Season with a pinch of salt and whisk to combine. Cover with cling film and chill for 15 minutes. To serve, divide the farro between four serving plates, top with the beetroot and lentils, and spoon over a dollop of yogurt.

150g (5½oz) uncooked farro

3 tbsp light olive oil

1 garlic clove, sliced

salt and freshly ground black pepper

250g (9oz) Greek yogurt

1 tbsp lemon juice

1 tsp lemon zest

1 small garlic clove, crushed

1 tbsp extra virgin olive oil

handful of flat-leaf parsley

For the lentils and vegetables

1 onion, finely sliced

3 garlic cloves, crushed

3 large beetroots, peeled and chopped into 3cm (1in) pieces

2 carrots, chopped into 2.5cm (1in) pieces

2 tsp tomato purée

100g (3½oz) black beluga lentils, rinsed and cleaned

200ml (7fl oz) good-quality red wine

250ml (9fl oz) vegetable stock

sprig each of rosemary and thyme

1 bay leaf

Make it vegan

Use a vegan yogurt alternative, such as coconut yogurt (see page 38), rather than greek yogurt.

Curries and Stir-fries

Curries and stir-fries are ideal flexitarian meals. From green lentil curry to quinoa cashew stir-fry and crispy fried tofu, these dishes are nutritious and full of flavour on their own, or simple to add dairy or meat to.

Chickpea Tikka Masala in Lettuce Cups

Creamy and surprisingly mild, the curry flavour in this dish is a wonderful match for the slightly sweet butterhead lettuce and the textured chickpeas.

serves 6   **prep** 20 mins   **cook** 30 mins

1. In a large frying pan, heat the ghee over a medium-low heat until shimmering. Add the white onion and cook for 2 minutes, or until soft. Add the garam masala, turmeric, chilli, and ginger. Cook for an additional minute to warm the spices.

2. Stir in the chickpeas, passata, and yogurt. Bring to the boil then reduce the heat to low and cook for 20 minutes, or until the sauce and chickpeas are completely warmed through. Season with salt and pepper to taste. Remove from the heat and let sit for 5 minutes.

3. To assemble, divide the chickpea mixture evenly among the leaves. Garnish with the red onion and coriander and serve immediately.

1 tbsp ghee

1 small white onion, chopped

1 tbsp garam masala

½ tsp turmeric

1 small green chilli, deseeded and finely chopped

¼ tsp grated fresh ginger

350g (12oz) cooked chickpeas

500ml (16fl oz) passata

50g (1¾oz) plain Greek-style yogurt

salt and freshly ground black pepper

12 leaves cos lettuce, washed and dried

60g (2oz) thinly sliced red onion

2 tbsp chopped coriander leaves

Why not try...

For texture and crunch, use Savoy cabbage instead of the lettuce.

Make it vegan

Replace the ghee with canola oil and the yogurt with coconut yogurt (see page 38).

Make it with meat

Add 125g (4½oz) cooked, chopped chicken breast along with the chickpeas in step 2.

Black Sesame and Coconut Curry Bowl

By themselves, shirataki noodles have very little taste, so pan-frying them in the curry sauce allows them to absorb all the gently spiced flavours of this simple vegan dish.

serves 4   **prep** 10 mins   **cook** 25 mins

1 In a medium, heavy-based saucepan, melt 2 tablespoons coconut oil over a medium heat. Add the onion and cook for 2 to 3 minutes until soft but not brown. Incorporate the garlic and ginger and cook for 1 minute more.

2 Add the red pepper and mushrooms and cook for 2 to 3 minutes until they start to deepen in colour. Add the remaining 1 tablespoon coconut oil, curry powder, and chilli powder (if using), and stir well to combine. Reduce the heat to low and cook for 1 minute until the spices release fragrance.

3 Incorporate the coconut milk and vegetable stock. Add the sweet potatoes and bring to the boil. Reduce to a simmer and cook, uncovered, for 10 to 12 minutes until the sweet potatoes are soft.

4 Meanwhile, bring a pan of water to the boil. Transfer the shirataki noodles to a colander and rinse thoroughly under cold running water for at least 30 seconds to rinse off the packaging liquid. In the pan of boiling water, cook the noodles for 2 minutes. Drain well, and set aside to cool completely.

5 Heat a large, non-stick frying pan over a high heat. Once cool, dry-fry the noodles for 2 minutes, stirring constantly. Add most of the sauce to the noodles and cook for another 2 minutes until the sauce is mostly absorbed.

6 Divide the noodles among 4 serving bowls and top with equal amounts of the curried vegetables and the remaining sauce. Garnish with equal amounts of the coriander, spring onions, and sesame seeds, and serve immediately.

3 tbsp coconut oil

½ red onion, finely chopped

2 garlic cloves, finely chopped

2.5cm (1in) piece fresh ginger root, finely chopped

½ large red pepper, diced

150g (5½oz) mushrooms, peeled and quartered

2 tsp curry powder

¼ tsp chilli powder (optional)

400ml can coconut milk

120ml (4fl oz) vegetable stock

300g (10oz) sweet potato, peeled and diced into 1cm (½in) cubes

2 × 200g packets shirataki or vermicelli noodles

handful of coriander leaves

2 spring onions, trimmed and sliced on the diagonal

½ tsp black sesame seeds

Make it with fish

Top each bowl with 4 cooked prawns before you serve.

Lentil and Broccoli Green Curry

The crunch of broccoli complements the creamy curry sauce, and the lentils introduce another layer of texture to this Thai dish, which is perfect over brown basmati or jasmine rice.

serves 8   **prep** 30 mins   **cook** 35 mins

1 In a large saucepan, warm the oil over a medium-low heat until shimmering. Add the shallot and garlic and cook for 2 minutes, or until soft. Add the curry paste and stir to combine. Cook for an additional minute.

2 Add the coconut milk, soy sauce, and makrut lime leaf or lime juice. Simmer for 10 minutes. Add the red pepper and cook for another 10 minutes, or until the pepper starts to become tender.

3 Stir in the broccoli, lentils, mushrooms, green beans, and basil. Cook for an additional 5–10 minutes, until the green beans and broccoli are tender and the mushrooms are cooked. Remove the makrut lime leaf, if using. Season with salt and pepper to taste. Serve immediately.

1 tbsp vegetable oil

1 shallot, finely chopped

1 garlic clove, finely chopped

1 tbsp green curry paste

400ml can coconut milk

½ tbsp soy sauce

1 makrut (kaffir) lime leaf or 1 tbsp fresh lime juice

1 small red pepper, deseeded and julienned

200g (7oz) broccoli florets

325g (11oz) cooked green lentils

100g (3½oz) shiitake mushrooms, sliced

75g (2½oz) chopped fresh green beans

1 tbsp finely chopped basil leaves

salt and freshly ground black pepper

Make it with meat

Add 225g (8oz) raw chicken breast, sliced, and cook with the shallots and garlic in step 1.

Curries and Stir-fries **173**

Thai Yellow Pumpkin Curry with Quinoa

This vibrant curry with its fresh, Thai flavours uses pumpkin and quinoa to create a hearty and warming supper that is really comforting in autumn or winter.

serves 4-6   **prep** 10 mins   **cook** 40 mins

1 Heat the oil in a large, lidded saucepan over a medium heat. Add the curry paste and onions and cook for 2 minutes, stirring frequently. Then add the pumpkin, coconut milk, stock, and quinoa to the pan. Bring to a simmer, cover, and cook for about 30 minutes.

2 Add the chickpeas and cook for 5 minutes or until the pumpkin is tender. Taste and adjust the seasoning as necessary. Remove from the heat. Garnish with coriander and serve immediately with lime wedges.

1 tbsp coconut oil or sunflower oil

3 tbsp Thai yellow curry paste

1 onion, finely chopped

1 pumpkin, about 800g (1¾lb), deseeded and chopped into bite-sized pieces

400ml can coconut milk

300ml (10fl oz) vegetable stock

200g (7oz) uncooked quinoa

400g can chickpeas, drained

salt and freshly ground black pepper

4 tbsp chopped coriander leaves, to garnish

2 limes, cut into wedges

Why not try...

You could try using sweet potato in place of the pumpkin, and garnish with flat-leaf parsley instead of the coriander.

Pigeon Pea Vindaloo

Characteristic of vindaloo, the high heat level in this Indian curry balances with warm spices, such as cinnamon and cardamom. Serve with rice or naan and some cooling yogurt raita.

serves 4   **prep** 25 mins   **cook** 35 mins

1   In a small bowl, combine the cumin, ground coriander, turmeric, cardamom, mustard, and paprika and stir thoroughly to combine.

2   In a heavy-bottomed pan, heat the oil over a medium heat until shimmering. Add the onion and cook for 3–4 minutes until it starts to become translucent.

3   Stir in the garlic, ginger, and chilli, and cook for an additional 2 minutes. Incorporate the spice mixture, bay leaf, cinnamon stick, passata, vinegar, and water, and bring to the boil. Reduce the heat and simmer, covered, for 10 minutes.

4   Add the pigeon peas (or black-eyed beans) and stir to combine. Bring to the boil then reduce to a simmer and cook, covered, for 20 minutes. Remove the cinnamon stick and bay leaf. Season with salt and pepper to taste. Serve immediately.

1¼ tbsp ground cumin

1 tbsp ground coriander

¾ tsp turmeric

⅔ tsp ground cardamom

½ tbsp ground mustard seeds

1 tbsp paprika

1 tbsp vegetable oil

1 small onion, diced

3 garlic cloves, finely chopped

¾ tbsp finely chopped fresh ginger

1 large hot red chilli, deseeded and finely chopped

1 bay leaf

1 cinnamon stick

225g (8oz) passata

1 tbsp red wine vinegar

240ml (8fl oz) water

450g (1lb) cooked pigeon peas or black-eyed beans

salt and freshly ground black pepper

Make it with meat

Brown 450g (1lb) chuck steak, diced, and add with the passata.

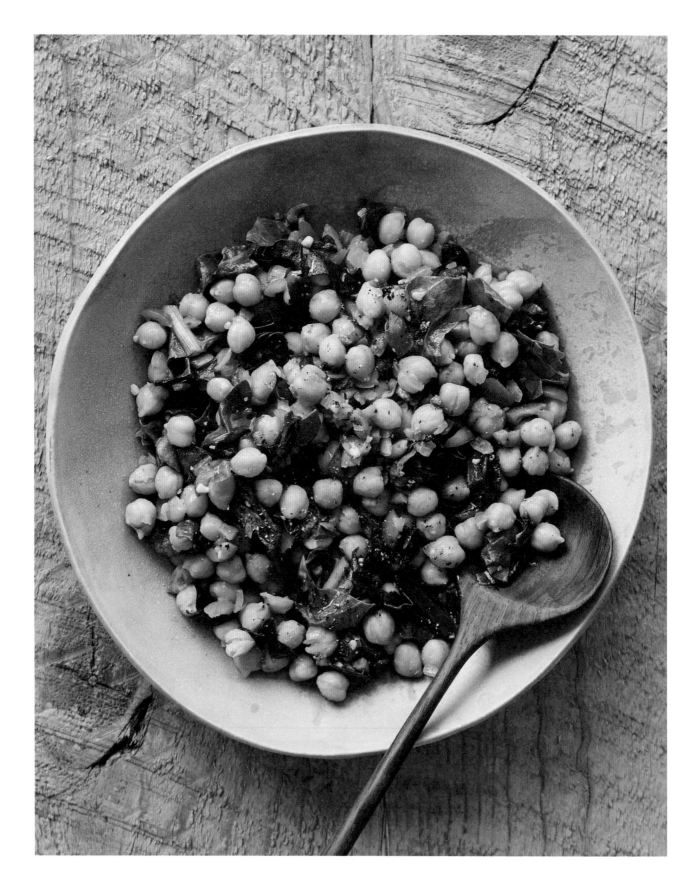

Braised Chickpeas with Preserved Lemon

A North African condiment, these lemon slices preserved in brine add a fragrant touch to a simply braised chickpea and chard recipe.

serves 6 **prep** 15 mins **cook** 35 mins

1 In a large flameproof casserole, warm the oil over a medium heat until shimmering. Add the onion and cook for 2 minutes, or until soft. Add the garlic and cook for an additional minute.

2 Add the chickpeas and Swiss chard and stir to combine. Add the stock and cook, covered, for 15 minutes, or until the chard begins to wilt.

3 Stir in the olives and preserved lemon. Cook, covered, for an additional 10 minutes. Season with salt and pepper to taste. Serve immediately.

1 tbsp olive oil

1 small onion, chopped

1 garlic clove, finely chopped

500g (1lb 2oz) cooked chickpeas

450g (1lb) chopped Swiss chard, leaves and stems

120ml (4fl oz) vegetable stock

75g (2½oz) chopped green olives

½ tbsp finely chopped preserved lemon, or zest and juice of 1 lemon

salt and freshly ground black pepper

Make it with meat

Finely dice 60g (2oz) pancetta and cook with the onion in step 1.

Cauliflower Curry

For this recipe, potatoes and cauliflower are tumbled in a tikka coconut sauce. This is a simple and economical dish to make, and can easily be made ahead and reheated when required.

serves 4-6 **prep** 15 mins **cook** 1 hr

1 Heat the oil in a large heavy-based pan over a medium heat, add the onion, and cook for 3-4 minutes until soft. Season with salt and pepper, stir through the ginger, garlic, and chillies, and cook for a couple of minutes. Stir in the tikka paste, chickpeas, coconut milk, and stock and bring to the boil. Reduce to a simmer and cook gently, partially covered with the lid and stirring occasionally, for 30 minutes.

2 Meanwhile, bring another large pan of salted water to the boil. Add the potatoes and cook for about 15 minutes or until just beginning to soften. Remove the potatoes with a slotted spoon and set aside. Put the cauliflower in the boiling water and cook for about 5 minutes, then drain well.

3 Tip the potato and cauliflower into the sauce and turn so they are well coated, then simmer very gently for a further 15 minutes or so, to allow all the flavours to mingle. Serve with some rice and naan.

1 tbsp vegetable oil

1 onion, roughly chopped

salt and freshly ground black pepper

5cm (2in) piece of fresh root ginger, peeled and finely chopped

3 garlic cloves, finely chopped

2 green chillies, deseeded and finely chopped

2 tbsp medium-hot tikka curry paste

400g can chickpeas, drained and rinsed

400ml can coconut milk

600ml (1 pint) hot vegetable stock

3 potatoes, peeled and cut into bite-sized pieces

1 cauliflower, cut into bite-sized florets

Paneer and Sweet Pepper Curry

The sweet peppers marry well with the paneer in this mild vegetarian curry. Paneer is an Indian cheese that won't melt upon cooking; you'll find it with the other cheeses at the supermarket.

serves 4-6 **prep** 20 mins **cook** 1 hr

1 Heat half the oil in a heavy-based pan over a medium-high heat, add the paneer and cook for 5-8 minutes, stirring, until golden all over. Remove and set aside.

2 Heat the remaining oil in the pan, add the ginger, chillies, curry leaves, cumin seeds, garam masala, and turmeric, and stir well to coat with the oil. Then add the peppers and cook over a low heat for about 15 minutes until beginning to soften.

3 Add the tomatoes and 100ml (3½fl oz) water and cook on low for 15 minutes. Return the paneer to the pan, season with salt and pepper, then simmer gently for 15-20 minutes, topping up with a little hot water if needed. Stir through the coriander and serve with rice, chapatis, or naan.

2 tbsp vegetable oil

230g packet paneer, cubed

10cm (4in) piece fresh root ginger, peeled and sliced

2 red chillies, deseeded and finely chopped

2 tbsp dried curry leaves, crushed

2 tsp cumin seeds

4 tsp garam masala

2 tsp ground turmeric

6 red peppers, deseeded and sliced

6 tomatoes, skinned and roughly chopped

salt and freshly ground black pepper

bunch of coriander, finely chopped

Make it vegan

Replace the paneer with the same amount of cubed firm tofu, and follow the same instructions in steps 1 and 3.

Courgette, Herb, and Lemon Tagine

Light, fresh, and zingy, this vegetarian version of a tagine is full of punchy flavours. It is a good dish to prepare ahead as the flavours improve with reheating.

serves 4   **prep** 25 mins   **cook** 45-55 mins

1 Heat half the oil in a large heavy-based pan or tagine over a low heat, add the onions, and cook for 8 minutes until soft and translucent. Season well with salt and pepper, then stir through the garlic, fennel seeds, cinnamon, harissa, and preserved lemons.

2 Add the tomatoes and stir well, crushing them with the back of a wooden spoon. Bring to the boil, then reduce to a simmer and cook over a low heat for 30-40 minutes. If the sauce starts to dry out, top up with a little hot water.

3 Cook the broccoli in a pan of boiling salted water for 3-5 minutes or until tender, then drain and refresh in cold water. Drain again and set aside. Heat the remaining oil in a frying pan over a low heat, add the courgettes and seasoning, and cook, stirring frequently, for 5 minutes or until they start to colour a little. Add the lemon juice and stir through the dill. Add the broccoli and courgettes to the sauce and stir through the parsley. Serve on warmed plates with couscous, lemon wedges, and a spoonful of harissa on the side.

2 tbsp olive oil

1 red onion, finely chopped

salt and freshly ground black pepper

3 garlic cloves, finely chopped

pinch of fennel seeds

pinch of ground cinnamon

1-2 tsp harissa paste, plus extra to serve

2 preserved lemons, quartered and flesh discarded

400g can whole tomatoes, chopped

1 head broccoli, broken into florets

3 courgettes, trimmed and sliced

juice of 1 lemon

handful of dill, finely chopped

handful of flat-leaf parsley, finely chopped

Miso Japanese Aubergine and Buckwheat Noodles

Japanese aubergines are long, thin, and have very few seeds, but you can also use any young aubergines you can find. With its umami flavour, this dish tastes light while being filling.

serves 4   **prep** 15 mins   **cook** 30 mins

1 Preheat the oven to 220°C (425°F/Gas 7). Lightly score the cut-side of the aubergines with the tip of a sharp knife to make a criss-cross design. Place cut-side down on a lightly oiled baking sheet and transfer to the top shelf of the oven. Bake for 10 to 15 minutes until soft.

2 Meanwhile, bring a large pan of salted water to the boil. To make the glaze: in a small saucepan, whisk together the miso paste and 4 tablespoons hot water. Then whisk in the mirin, sugar, and sesame oil. Bring briefly to the boil, whisking constantly until the sugar has dissolved. Remove from the heat and set aside.

3 Cook the noodles in the boiling water according to the package instructions until just al dente, then drain and rinse briefly under cold water. Toss with a drizzle of sesame oil to prevent sticking.

4 When the aubergine is soft, remove from the oven and turn the oven on to a high grill setting. Line the baking sheet with foil and arrange the aubergines cut-side up on the sheet. Brush the cut-sides with the glaze. Return to the top shelf of the oven and grill until well browned and crisp on top, about 10 minutes. Remove the aubergines from the oven occasionally to brush with more glaze when it has been absorbed (about 3 times). Sprinkle with the sesame seeds and grill for one last time until the sesame seeds are brown.

5 Heat the sunflower oil in a wok over a medium heat. Add the cabbage and bean sprouts and stir-fry for 1 minute. Stir the soy sauce into the remaining glaze. Add the noodles, spring onions, and glaze to the wok and cook for 1 minute more until heated through. Add the coriander and toss well to combine. Divide among 4 serving dishes, and top each with 2 pieces of aubergine. Garnish with coriander leaves and serve immediately.

2 firm Japanese or other young aubergines, trimmed and halved lengthways, then in half widthways

salt

225g (8oz) buckwheat soba noodles

sesame oil, to toss

1 tbsp sesame seeds

1 tbsp sunflower oil, plus extra for greasing

175g (6oz) very finely sliced green cabbage

175g (6oz) bean sprouts

1 tbsp soy sauce

4 large spring onions, trimmed and very finely

2 tbsp chopped coriander leaves, plus whole leaves to garnish

For the glaze

2 tbsp white miso paste

4 tbsp mirin

1½ tbsp sugar

2 tsp sesame oil

Make it with fish

Add 400g (14oz) skinned, cubed salmon to the wok in step 5 before the cabbage, and cook for 2–3 minutes.

Quinoa Cashew Stir-Fry with Chilli and Lime Sauce

This simple stir-fry is light, yet full of flavour and colour. The lime gives it an added zing that pairs well with the sweetness of the toasted cashews and crunchy vegetables.

serves 2   **prep** 20 mins   **cook** 20 mins

1 Place the quinoa in a large saucepan. Cover with 125ml (4¼fl oz) of water and simmer for about 10 minutes or until all the water has been absorbed. Then remove from the heat and set aside.

2 Heat a large wok or frying pan over a high heat. Add the cashew nuts and toast until lightly coloured. Remove from the heat and roughly chop. Add the oil to the pan. Then add the carrots, cabbage, bean sprouts, and onions. Cook, stirring frequently, for about 5 minutes or until lightly cooked.

3 Meanwhile, for the sauce, place all the ingredients in a bowl and mix to combine. Add the quinoa to the vegetables and mix well. Pour over the chilli and lime sauce, mix well, and cook for 1–2 minutes. Remove from the heat and serve hot.

100g (3½oz) uncooked quinoa

50g (1¾oz) cashew nuts

2 tbsp light olive oil

115g (4oz) carrot, roughly chopped

115g (4oz) cabbage, roughly chopped

100g (3½oz) bean sprouts

85g (3oz) red onion, thinly sliced

For the sauce

juice of 1 lime and grated zest of ½ lime

2 tbsp soy sauce

2 tbsp honey

1 red chilli, deseeded and finely chopped

Make it with meat

Chop 200g (7oz) chicken breast into slices and cook with the vegetables in step 2.

Poblanos Stuffed with Spicy Sorghum and Black Bean Stir-Fry

Green poblano peppers have a sweet and mild heat that makes them the perfect companion for this well-spiced sorghum stir-fry. An impressive dish, it's also easy to make.

serves 6   **prep** 10 mins, plus cooling   **cook** 1 hr 20 mins

1. Place the sorghum and stock in a small, lidded saucepan and bring to the boil. Then reduce to a simmer, cover, and cook for about 45 minutes. Remove from the heat and leave, covered, for a further 10 minutes. Then drain any remaining water and set aside.

2. Meanwhile, preheat the oven to 230°C (450°F/Gas 8). Place the poblano peppers on a lined baking sheet. Brush with half of the oil and season with salt and pepper. Place in the oven and roast for 15–20 minutes, until they start to brown and are tender. Remove from the heat and leave to cool slightly. Once cool enough to handle, slit the peppers in the centre, lengthways, and remove the seeds.

3. Heat the remaining oil in a large cast-iron pan over a medium heat. Add the onions and sauté for 5–8 minutes or until softened. Then add the garlic, chilli powder, oregano, cumin, and cayenne pepper. Mix to combine and cook for 2–3 minutes, stirring frequently.

4. Add the sorghum, beans, and tomatoes and stir to combine. Cook for 5 minutes, stirring occasionally. Then add the corn and cook for a further 2–3 minutes. Taste, and adjust the seasoning if needed. Spoon the stir-fry mixture into the poblano peppers and scatter any extra on the plates. Garnish with Cheddar and serve immediately.

100g (3½oz) uncooked sorghum (found in health food or African food stores)

500ml (16fl oz) vegetable stock

6 large poblano peppers

2 tbsp sunflower oil

salt and freshly ground black pepper

1 small red onion, roughly chopped

3 garlic cloves, crushed

1 tsp chilli powder

1 tsp oregano

½ tsp ground cumin

¼ tsp cayenne pepper

400g can black beans, drained and rinsed

150g (5½oz) plum tomatoes, deseeded and diced

150g can corn kernels

1 tbsp freshly grated Cheddar cheese, to serve

Make it vegan

Use a plant-based cheese alternative or nut cheese (see page 37) instead of Cheddar.

Sesame-crusted Tofu with Green Beans and Black Rice

This vegetarian dish uses sesame seeds in place of breadcrumbs to coat tender tofu, giving it a crunchy, nutty texture, and pairs it with a spicy, salty green bean stir-fry.

serves 4   **prep** 15 mins   **cook** 50 mins

1 Place the rice in a large saucepan and cook according to packet instructions. Remove from the heat, cover, and set aside. Pat the tofu dry with kitchen paper and cut 16 × 2.5cm (1in) thick triangles. Set aside.

2 Place the cornflour and sesame seeds in a shallow dish and mix to combine. Place the egg in a small bowl. Season the tofu with salt and pepper and brush lightly with the egg. Then toss the tofu in the cornflour mixture until lightly coated.

3 Heat the grapeseed oil in a large frying pan over a medium-low heat. Once the oil has heated, reduce the heat to low and add the tofu. Cook for 3–4 minutes on each side, turning the tofu gently to prevent it breaking apart, until evenly browned on each side. Remove with a slotted spoon, set aside on a lined plate, and keep warm. Drain the excess oil from the pan.

4 Add the sesame oil to the pan and increase the heat to medium. Add the onions, ginger, and chillies. Cook for about 5 minutes, stirring frequently, until softened. Then add the garlic and cook for another minute. Add the green beans and cook, stirring, for 3–4 minutes.

5 Add the tamari sauce and spring onions. Season with pepper and cook, stirring, for about 3 minutes. Add the tofu and gently heat through for 2 minutes. Do not stir the tofu as it may break apart. Remove from the heat. Divide the rice between four serving plates. Top with the green bean and onion stir-fry and the tofu. Sprinkle over sesame seeds, drizzle with some oil and tamari sauce, and serve warm.

300g black rice

400g (14oz) extra firm tofu, drained

4 tbsp cornflour

4 tbsp sesame seeds, plus extra to serve

1 egg, lightly beaten

salt and freshly ground black pepper

2–3 tbsp grapeseed oil

2 tbsp sesame oil, plus extra to serve

1 onion, thinly sliced

1 tsp grated fresh root ginger

3 mild red chillies, deseeded and sliced into 1cm (½in) pieces

3 garlic cloves, crushed and thinly sliced

200g (7oz) green beans, blanched

1 tbsp tamari sauce, plus extra to serve

2 spring onions, cut into 2.5cm (1in) long pieces

Make it vegan

Use 3 tbsp aquafaba in place of the egg. Lightly beat it with a whisk and use it as you would the egg in step 2.

Baked Dishes and Casseroles

Satisfy your craving for hearty meals with these casseroles and baked dishes. From lasagne to enchiladas, you'll find easy weeknight dinners to enjoy when the weather starts to cool.

Creamy Fontina and Truffle Lasagne

The sweet, creamy fontina and truffle oil make this an especially luxurious lasagne. The buttery sauce is delicious with a sharp green salad to balance the richness of the dish.

serves 6   **prep** 20 mins   **cook** 1 hr, plus standing

1   Preheat the oven to 200°C (400°F/Gas 6). To make the filling: in a large frying pan, heat the olive oil over a high heat. Working in two batches, partially cook the mushrooms for 3 to 4 minutes, turning often. Recombine the batches and add the garlic. Cook for 1 minute more.

2   Add the artichokes and truffle oil. Season well with salt and pepper. Stir, then set aside to cool.

3   To make the sauce: in a heavy-based saucepan, melt the butter over a medium heat. Remove from the heat and whisk in the rice flour. Gradually whisk in the milk. Return the pan to the heat and cook, whisking constantly, for 2 to 3 minutes until the mixture thickens and starts to boil. Reduce the heat to low and continue to cook for 2 to 3 minutes, whisking occasionally. Finally, add two-thirds of the cheese, and whisk until melted. Remove from the heat and season well with salt and pepper.

4   To assemble the lasagne: in a 23 × 33cm (9 × 13in) baking dish, spread one-quarter of the sauce to coat the bottom of the dish. On top of that, layer one-third of the filling, and a single layer of lasagne sheets. Then layer with another one-quarter of the sauce, one-third of the filling, and a single layer of lasagne sheets. Top with another one-quarter of the sauce, the remaining mushroom mixture, and a final layer of lasagne sheets.

5   Cover the top with the remaining sauce and remaining cheese. Transfer to the middle shelf of the oven and bake for 40 to 45 minutes until well browned and cooked through. Leave to stand for 10 to 15 minutes before cutting and serving.

2 tbsp olive oil

450g (1lb) cleaned, trimmed, and roughly chopped mixed mushrooms (such as cremini, portobello, oyster, and shiitake)

1 large garlic clove, crushed

340g jar grilled artichoke halves in oil, drained and roughly chopped

2 tsp truffle oil

salt and freshly ground black pepper

8–10 fresh lasagne sheets (see p33)

For the sauce

60g (2oz) unsalted butter

60g (2oz) sweet white rice flour

550ml (18fl oz) whole milk

140g (5oz) fontina cheese (or mozzerella), roughly grated

Make it vegan

Replace the sauce in this recipe with vegan Béchamel Sauce (see page 42). Top the lasagne with a plant-based mozzerella in step 5.

Curried Black Lentil Stuffed Onions

The nuttiness of black lentils and quinoa mixed with creamy goat's cheese makes these onions a unique main course.

serves 8   **prep** 30 mins   **cook** 1 hr

1 Preheat the oven to 190°C (375°F). Trim both ends off the onions and discard the skins. Cut each onion horizontally in half to create 2 flat sections. To create a well for the filling, with a spoon or melon baller gently scoop out the middle of each onion half, leaving the bottom of the onion intact.

2 Arrange the onions in a 20 × 20cm (8 × 8in) baking dish, well-side up, and fill the bottom of the dish with water. Cover the dish with foil and bake for 40 minutes, or until the onions are tender.

3 Meanwhile, in a medium saucepan, combine the stock, curry powder, and garam masala. Bring gradually to the boil and add the dry quinoa. Return to the boil then reduce to a simmer and cook, covered, for 15–18 minutes until tender. Remove from the heat and let sit, covered, for 5 minutes.

4 In a large mixing bowl, combine the cooked and seasoned quinoa, black lentils, goat's cheese, and 10g (¼oz) coriander. Thoroughly combine. Season with salt and pepper to taste.

5 Spoon an equal amount of quinoa mixture into each onion half. Bake, uncovered, for 20 minutes, or until the filling is toasted and warmed through. Garnish with the remaining 2 tablespoons of coriander and serve immediately.

4 onions

240ml (8fl oz) water

550ml (18fl oz) vegetable stock

½ tsp curry powder

½ tsp garam masala

175g (6oz) uncooked red, black, and white quinoa

140g (5oz) cooked black lentils

175g (6oz) crumbled goat's cheese

10g (¼oz) plus 2 tbsp chopped coriander leaves

salt and freshly ground black pepper

Make it vegan

Replace the goat's cheese with a nut cheese (see page 37).

Make it with meat

Reduce the cooked black lentils to 100g (3½oz) and add 225g (8oz) cooked minced lamb along with the lentils.

Moth Bean Stuffed Sweet Potatoes

The surprising mix of sweet and savoury in these baked potatoes makes for a truly luscious meal or hearty side dish.

makes 8   **prep** 15 mins   **cook** 1 hr 15 mins

1   Preheat the oven to 220°C (425°F) and line a baking tray with foil.

2   Cut each potato in half lengthways. Lightly oil each cut side. Arrange the potatoes cut-side down on the baking tray and bake for 30–40 minutes until tender all the way through.

3   To assemble, turn the sweet potato halves cut-side up. With a fork, fluff the inside of the potatoes while keeping the skin intact. Top each potato half with an equal amount of moth beans (or lentils) and an equal amount of Brie. Season with salt and pepper.

4   Bake for an additional 8–10 minutes until the Brie is melted and gooey. Sprinkle each potato half with 2 tablespoons of pomegranate seeds and 2 tablespoons of chopped coriander. Serve immediately.

4 sweet potatoes, about 1kg (2lb) in total

500g (1lb 2oz) cooked moth beans, or black lentils

225g (8oz) Brie cheese

salt and freshly ground black pepper

175g (6oz) pomegranate seeds

30g (1oz) roughly chopped coriander leaves

Make it with meat

Crumble 60g (2oz) cooked crispy bacon into each potato, along with the pomegranate seeds.

Baked Lentil Spaghetti Squash

For infusing your diet with complex carbohydrates, spaghetti squash is a healthy alternative to pasta. Each squash half is its own nutty, casserole-type dish in a self-contained serving.

serves 2   **prep** 25 mins   **cook** 45 mins

1 Preheat the oven to 190°C (375°F). Cut the spaghetti squash in half lengthways and use a spoon to scrape the seeds out of each half. Drizzle each half with 1 tablespoon of oil, and arrange cut-side down on a baking tray. Cook for 30–35 minutes until tender but not mushy.

2 Meanwhile, in a medium mixing bowl, combine the lentils, walnuts, thyme, and lemon zest. Set aside until the squash is cooked.

3 With a fork, scrape the squash flesh to expose and fluff the spaghetti shreds. Season with salt and pepper. Divide the lentil filling evenly between the halves and crumble goat's cheese over each. Bake for an additional 10 minutes, or until the cheese softens. Serve immediately, directly from the squash shell.

1 spaghetti squash (available from farmers' markets throughout winter and spring)

2 tbsp olive oil

450g (1lb) cooked green or Puy lentils

60g (2oz) walnuts, toasted and roughly chopped

1 tbsp thyme leaves

zest of 1 lemon

salt and freshly ground black pepper

115g (4oz) soft goat's cheese

Make it vegan

Omit the goat's cheese, or use a nut cheese (see page 37).

Make it with meat

Reduce the lentils to 225g (8oz) and add 130g (4½oz) cooked, seasoned minced turkey to the filling.

Butter Bean Enchiladas

Tomatillos are a staple in Mexican sauces. Their tart, fruity flavour shines in this herby enchilada sauce, wonderfully set off by buttery beans and a sweet medley of vegetables.

makes 10   **prep** 55 mins   **cook** 1 hr

1 Preheat the oven to 180°C (350°F). On a lightly oiled baking tray, arrange the tomatillos, jalapeños, and onion. Roast for 20–25 minutes until tender. Leave to cool slightly. To make the sauce, transfer the roasted vegetables to a blender and combine with the coriander sprigs and stock. Blend until completely smooth. Season with salt and pepper.

2 To make the filling, in a large frying pan heat the oil over a medium-low heat. Add the garlic and cook for 1–2 minutes until soft. Add the courgettes and sweetcorn and cook, covered, for an additional 2–3 minutes until the courgette starts to become tender. Stir in the spinach, cumin, coriander, and dried chillies. Cover and cook for another 3–4 minutes until the spinach wilts slightly. Stir in the butter beans. Season with salt and pepper to taste. Remove from the heat and leave to cool slightly.

3 Lightly oil a 23 × 30cm (9 × 12in) glass or ceramic baking dish. Lightly coat the bottom with sauce. To assemble, work with one tortilla at a time on a clean, flat work surface. Place 4 tablespoons of filling onto the tortilla and top with 1½–2 tablespoons of grated cheese. Roll tightly and place seam-side down in the dish. Repeat to make 10 enchiladas in total.

4 Top the enchiladas with the remaining sauce. Sprinkle the remaining cheese over the top. Cover with foil and bake for 15 minutes. Uncover and bake for another 10 minutes, or until the cheese melts. Garnish with chopped coriander and serve immediately.

675g (1½lb) tomatillos, husks removed, roughly chopped (or small, unripe tomatoes, roughly chopped)

2 medium jalapeños, deseeded and chopped

1 onion, chopped

30g (1oz) sprigs of coriander

175ml (6fl oz) vegetable stock

salt and freshly ground black pepper

1 tbsp vegetable oil

1 garlic clove, finely chopped

2 courgettes, diced

150g (5½oz) fresh sweetcorn kernels

175g (6oz) baby spinach

1½ tsp ground cumin

1 tsp ground coriander

pinch of crushed dried chillies

225g (8oz) cooked butter beans

10 small corn tortillas

225g (8oz) mozzarella cheese

15g (½oz) chopped coriander leaves

Why not try...

Use crumbled feta instead of grated cheese. Place 1 tablespoon inside each enchilada and sprinkle the rest on top.

Make it vegan

Use a nut cheese instead of mozzarella (see page 37).

Make it with meat

Omit one courgette and add 125g (4½oz) cooked, chopped chicken or pork to the filling.

Pigeon Pea Samosa Bake

Filled with the unique aromas and flavours of Indian spiced potatoes and pigeon peas, this casserole with its crunchy filo topping is a nod to traditional samosa pastry.

serves 8   **prep** 30 mins   **cook** 45 mins

1 Preheat the oven to 180°C (350°F). Lightly oil a 23cm (9in) round baking dish.

2 Bring a large saucepan of water to a rapid boil. Add the potatoes and cook for 8-10 minutes until tender to the point of a knife. Meanwhile, place the green peas in a sieve or colander. When the potatoes are cooked, pour the potatoes and hot water over the peas. Let drain thoroughly.

3 In a large frying pan, heat 2 tablespoons of ghee over a medium-low heat until shimmering. Add the onion and chilli and cook for 2-3 minutes until soft. Incorporate the ginger, ground coriander, garam masala, cumin, turmeric, cayenne, curry powder, and water. Cook for an additional minute until the spices are warmed through.

4 Add the potatoes and green peas, pigeon peas (or black-eyed beans), stock, chopped coriander, and remaining 1 tablespoon ghee. Stir to combine. Season with salt and pepper to taste. Remove from the heat.

5 Transfer the mixture to the baking dish. Crinkle the filo sheet and place atop the potato mixture. Bake for 20-25 minutes until the filo pastry is golden brown, then serve.

550g (1¼lb) peeled and diced potatoes

115g (4oz) frozen green peas, thawed

3 tbsp ghee

1 small onion, diced

1 small green chilli, deseeded and finely chopped

¼ tsp ground ginger

¼ tsp ground coriander

¾ tsp garam masala

1 tsp ground cumin

¼ tsp turmeric

¼ tsp ground cayenne pepper

¾ tsp curry powder

1 tbsp water

75g (2½oz) cooked pigeon peas or black-eyed beans

90ml (3fl oz) vegetable stock

10g (¼oz) chopped coriander leaves

4 sheets of frozen filo pastry, thawed

Why not try...

For an aromatic garnish, sprinkle the pastry with crushed cumin seeds before baking.

Make it vegan

Replace the ghee with canola oil.

Make it with meat

Add 125g (4½oz) cooked, seasoned minced lamb with the peas in step 4

Ratatouille Casserole with Farro and Feta

A mix of baked Mediterranean vegetables, tomato sauce, and tender farro is topped with contrasting salty feta cheese for a warm and filling meal that is perfect at any time of the year.

serves 4   **prep** 10 mins, plus overnight soaking   **cook** 1 hr 30 mins

1   Place the farro in a large bowl, cover with water, and leave to soak overnight or for up to 8 hours. Then drain any remaining water, rinse under running water, and drain well again. Set aside.

2   Preheat the oven to 180°C (350°F/Gas 4). Place the aubergine cubes in a colander, sprinkle with the salt, and press down with a heavy object. Leave to draw out the water and any bitterness.

3   Place the peppers, courgette, onions, and aubergine in a 2 litre (3½ pint) casserole. Spread them out evenly and drizzle with the oil. Add the farro to the dish and toss lightly to mix with the vegetables.

4   Place the tomatoes, stock, rosemary, and garlic in a large bowl and mix to combine. Add the mixture to the casserole and mix well. Cover, place in the oven, and bake for 1 hour and 15 minutes or until the vegetables are tender and the farro is cooked.

5   Remove from the heat, take off the lid, and sprinkle over the feta. Return to the oven, uncovered, and cook for about 15 minutes or until the feta starts to turn golden. Remove from the heat and season to taste if needed. Garnish with basil and serve hot.

100g (3½oz) uncooked farro

1 aubergine, cut into cubes

½ tsp salt

2 red or orange peppers, deseeded and cut into bite-sized pieces

1 courgette, cut into bite-sized pieces

1 red onion, finely chopped

1 tbsp light olive oil

400g can chopped tomatoes

250ml (9fl oz) vegetable stock

¼ tsp dried rosemary

1 garlic clove, finely chopped

200g (7oz) feta cheese, crumbled

2 tsp chopped basil leaves, to serve

Make it vegan

Omit the feta cheese or replace it with a nut cheese (see page 37).

Pasta and Grains

Pasta and grain dishes are simple to prepare and make the perfect flexitarian meal – you can easily substitute ingredients to meet your dietary requirements.

Shaved Asparagus, Mint and Edamame Spaghetti

This vibrant green sauce is perfect for a light meal. Mint provides an unexpected and refreshing flavour that is delicious served with the tender asparagus and edamame.

serves 4 **prep** 10 mins **cook** 20 mins

1 Bring a large pan of salted water to the boil. To prepare the asparagus, place each spear flat on a chopping board and use a peeler to shave into very thin slices.

2 Cook the edamame in the boiling water for 1 minute. Remove with a slotted spoon and put into a bowl of iced water.

3 Add the pasta to the boiling water and cook according to the package instructions until just al dente. When the pasta is cooked, drain and reserve 120ml (4fl oz) cooking water. Set the pasta aside.

4 Meanwhile, when the spaghetti is nearly cooked, heat the olive oil in a large, non-stick frying pan. Add the asparagus and leek and cook for 2 minutes, stirring frequently, until the asparagus starts to soften. Add the garlic and edamame and cook for 1 minute more. Remove from the heat.

5 Add the ricotta and 4 tablespoons of the reserved cooking water to the pasta pan. Whisk until smooth, adding more cooking water as necessary. Add the asparagus mixture to the pan and mix together over a low heat.

6 Return the spaghetti to the pan, along with the mint and Parmesan. Toss well. Season well with salt and pepper. Divide among 4 serving plates and serve immediately with more Parmesan, mint leaves, and a drizzle of olive oil on top.

salt and freshly ground black pepper

225g (8oz) large asparagus, trimmed

115g (4oz) frozen shelled edamame

400g (14oz) dried wholemeal spaghetti

2 tbsp olive oil, plus extra to serve

1 large leek, white parts only, trimmed and julienned

1 large garlic clove, crushed

115g (4oz) ricotta cheese

1 large handful of fresh mint leaves, finely chopped, plus extra whole leaves to garnish

2 tbsp grated Parmesan cheese, plus extra to serve

Make it vegan

Instead of the ricotta, put 115g (4oz) firm tofu, 2 tbsp lemon juice, 1 tbsp nutritional yeast, and 1 tbsp extra virgin olive oil in a blender and pulse until it is semi-puréed. Use this tofu mixture as per the ricotta in step 5. Omit the Parmesan cheese or use a vegan alternative.

Roasted Cauliflower and Mint Orecchiette

The hearty yet delicately shaped pasta is a perfect partner for creamy roasted cauliflower and light, fresh herbs. If you can't find yellow cauliflower, substitute with white cauliflower.

serves 4   **prep** 5 mins   **cook** 20 mins

1 Preheat the oven to 200°C (400°F/Gas 6). Bring a large pan of salted water to the boil. To prepare the cauliflower: in a large bowl, mix the olive oil, garlic, and red pepper flakes. Season with salt and pepper to taste. Add the cauliflower and toss with your hands, making sure the seasoning is rubbed in well.

2 Evenly spread the cauliflower in a large, metal roasting pan. Transfer to the top shelf of the oven and roast for 15 minutes, or until just cooked and browned in places.

3 Meanwhile, cook the orecchiette in the boiling water according to the package instructions until just al dente. Drain and reserve 240ml (8fl oz) cooking water.

4 In a large, cast-iron frying pan, melt the butter and olive oil over a medium heat. Add about 2 tablespoons cooking water and allow to bubble. Add the orecchiette and cook for 1 to 2 minutes until the pasta has absorbed most of the liquid.

5 Gently toss the cauliflower in the pasta. (Be sure to include all the crispy bits of garlic and red pepper flakes from the roasting pan.) Transfer to 4 serving dishes and top with equal amounts of the parsley and mint. Serve immediately with Parmesan.

salt and freshly ground black pepper

400g (14oz) dried orecchiette

2 tbsp unsalted butter

2 tbsp olive oil

2 tbsp finely chopped flat-leaf parsley

2 tbsp mint

grated Parmesan cheese, to serve

For the cauliflower

4 tbsp olive oil

2 garlic cloves, crushed

1 tsp red pepper flakes

450g (1lb) yellow (or white) cauliflower florets

Make it vegan

Replace the butter with a vegetable oil spread and the cheese with a plant-based Parmesan.

Sweet Potato Gnocchi and Hazelnut Gremolata

The zesty flavour and crunchy texture of the hazelnut gremolata contrasts well with the soft, slightly sweet gnocchi. Creamy, rich cheese sauce makes this dish truly decadent.

serves 4–6 **prep** 40 mins **cook** 1 hr 20 mins, plus cooling

1 Preheat the oven to 230°C (450°F/Gas 8). To make the gnocchi dough: wash and dry the sweet potatoes. Cut a small slit in the skins. Place in the oven and bake for 45 minutes, or until fork-tender. Remove from the oven and leave to cool completely.

2 Cut the cooled potatoes in half. Scoop the flesh into a medium bowl and mash with a potato masher. Stir in the sage and Parmesan, and season with salt and pepper. Stir in the sweet rice flour, millet flour, and almond flour, mixing together well to form a soft, sticky dough.

3 To shape the gnocchi: place the dough onto a work surface lightly dusted with flour. Cut the dough into 4 sections and work with 1 section at a time, keeping the rest covered with cling film. With your hands, roll a section of dough into a long, thin cylinder, about 2.5cm (1in) wide. Cut the cylinder into discs about 2cm (³/₄in) thick. Roll each disc into a small ball in your hands, then place on the work surface and tap to flatten slightly. When all are shaped, run the tines of a fork over the tops of the gnocchi to make indentations.

4 To make the gremolata: in a non-stick frying pan, dry-fry the hazelnuts over a medium heat for 2 minutes, stirring frequently, until golden brown in places. Remove from the heat. Once cool, rub them well in a clean tea towel to remove as much of the skins as possible. Set aside to cool, then finely chop.

5 Bring a large pan of salted water to the boil. In a small bowl, mix together the hazelnuts, parsley, lemon zest, and Parmesan. Season well with black pepper.

6 Reduce the boiling water to a simmer. Working in batches, add the gnocchi to the water and cook for 4 to 5 minutes until they float to the surface. Remove with a slotted spoon and place on a plate lined with kitchen paper to absorb the water. Continue until all are cooked.

7 To make the cheese sauce: add the cream and grated cheese to a small saucepan. Scatter the sweet rice flour over the surface and whisk in. Slowly bring to the boil, stirring constantly, until the sauce thickens and starts to bubble. Reduce the heat to low and cook for 1 minute more until thick and smooth. Season with black pepper.

8 Grease a large, shallow, ovenproof dish. Arrange the gnocchi in an even layer in the dish. Spread the cheese sauce over the top. Transfer to the top shelf of the oven and bake, uncovered, for 10 to 12 minutes until the top is golden brown and crispy. Remove from the oven and leave to cool for 5 to 10 minutes. Scatter the top with the hazelnut gremolata before serving.

For the gnocchi dough

2 medium sweet potatoes, about 300g (10oz) in total

1 tsp very finely chopped sage leaves

30g (1oz) finely grated Parmesan cheese

salt and freshly ground black pepper

60g (2oz) sweet rice flour

60g (2oz) millet flour

60g (2oz) almond flour

For the gremolata

15g (½oz) hazelnuts, roughly chopped

1 tbsp finely chopped flat-leaf parsley

½ tsp lemon zest

1 tbsp freshly grated Parmesan cheese

For the cheese sauce

120ml (4fl oz) double cream

115g (4oz) grated cheese, such as Gruyère or fontina

1 tsp sweet rice flour

Citrus Courgette Cannelloni with Goat's Cheese

Griddling the courgette slices helps them to become soft and easy to roll. The lightly charred flavour is a nice addition to the cheesy and lemony filling. Serve with a crisp green salad.

serves 4   **prep** 15 mins   **cook** 40 mins, plus cooling

1 Heat a cast-iron griddle pan and lightly brush with olive oil. Griddle the courgette slices for 1 to 2 minutes on each side until soft and lightly marked with grill marks. At the same time, in a non-stick frying pan, dry-fry the pine nuts over a medium heat for 2 to 3 minutes, turning frequently, until golden brown. Set aside to cool. Blot any excess moisture with kitchen paper once cool.

2 In a small bowl, beat together the goat's cheese, basil, lemon zest, and pine nuts. Season well with salt and pepper.

3 To assemble the cannelloni: portion a large, walnut-sized spoonful of goat's cheese mixture and place on the courgette slice. Spread out the cheese along the length of the slice. Roll the slice up. Place in a lightly oiled shallow ovenproof dish. Repeat to assemble the remaining cannelloni.

4 Preheat the oven to 230°C (450°F/Gas 8). To make the cheese sauce: in a small saucepan, melt the butter over a medium heat. Remove from the heat and whisk in the rice flour. Continue to whisk, slowly adding in the milk. Return to the heat and slowly bring to the boil, whisking frequently, until the mixture thickens. Reduce the heat to low and continue to cook for 2 to 3 minutes. Season well with salt and pepper and add most of the grated cheese, reserving some to sprinkle over the top. Whisk the sauce until the cheese melts, adding more milk if needed to help achieve a pourable consistency. Remove from the heat.

5 Pour the sauce over the cannelloni and top with the remaining grated cheese. Transfer to the top shelf of the oven. Cook, uncovered, for 15 to 20 minutes until the top is golden brown and the cannelloni are cooked through. Remove from the oven and leave to cool for 10 minutes, or until the cheese settles. Garnish with the basil and a drizzle of olive oil, and serve.

olive oil, for greasing and to serve

2 fat courgettes, about 300g (10oz) each, trimmed and cut into 12 thin slices lengthways with a mandoline

60g (2oz) pine nuts

200g (7oz) soft goat's cheese, room temperature

2 tbsp finely chopped basil, plus whole leaves to garnish

zest of 1 small or ½ large lemon

salt and freshly ground black pepper

For the cheese sauce

15g (½oz) unsalted butter

15g (½oz) sweet rice flour

100ml (3½fl oz) whole milk

30g (1oz) strong cheese, such as Cheddar, grated

Make it vegan

Use a nut cheese (see page 37) in place of the goat's cheese. And replace the cheese sauce with vegan Béchamel Sauce (see page 42), adding in 30g (1oz) plant-based cheese if you'd like.

Rainbow Lentil Meatballs with Arrabbiata Sauce

Lentil meatballs and spicy tomato sauce are a vegetarian alternative to the comfort food classic, loaded with protein and fibre. Serve with pasta or bread and Parmesan cheese.

serves 18 **prep** 15 mins **cook** 40 mins

1 Preheat the oven to 180°C (350°F). Lightly oil a baking tray. In a large mixing bowl, combine the red and brown lentils, egg, breadcrumbs, garlic powder, oregano, lemon zest, and cayenne.

2 With your hands, form approximately 1 tablespoon of the lentil mixture into a meatball and place on the baking tray. Repeat with the remaining mixture. Bake for 25 minutes, rotating the meatballs halfway through.

3 Meanwhile, to make the arrabbiata sauce, in a saucepan warm the oil over a medium-low heat. Add the onion and cook for 2 minutes, or until soft. Add the tomatoes and chillies. Simmer over a low heat for 15 minutes, or until the sauce is warmed through. Season with salt and pepper to taste.

4 Serve the meatballs with cooked spaghetti, topped with the sauce.

300g (10oz) cooked red lentils, thoroughly drained

85g (3oz) cooked brown lentils, thoroughly drained

1 large egg, lightly beaten

45g (1½oz) panko breadcrumbs

½ tsp garlic powder

1 tsp dried oregano

zest of 1 large lemon

¼ tsp ground cayenne pepper

2 tbsp olive oil

1 small onion, finely chopped

2 × 400g (14oz) cans chopped tomatoes

1 tbsp crushed dried chillies

salt and freshly ground black pepper

Make it vegan

Replace the egg with 3 tbsp aquafaba.

Make it with meat

Add 225g (8oz) minced beef or crumbled Italian sausage along with the onion in step 3.

Three Bean Paella

This colourful twist on the classic Spanish dish features a trio of meaty pulses in addition to saffron-scented rice, roasted red peppers, and tangy green olives.

serves 10   **prep** 35 mins   **cook** 1 hr 5 mins

1 In a 25cm (10in) paella pan or large cast-iron frying pan, warm the oil over a medium heat until shimmering. Add the onion and cook for 2 minutes, or until it starts to soften. Stir in the garlic and cook for 30 seconds, or until fragrant. Incorporate the saffron, dried chillies, tomatoes, and paprika. Stir in the rice and cook for 2–3 minutes.

2 Add the stock to the rice mixture and stir. Bring to the boil then reduce the heat to low and cook, covered, for 20 minutes. Stir in the haricot beans, pigeon peas (or black-eyed beans), and kidney beans. Cover again and cook for an additional 10 minutes. Scatter the green peas across the top and cook without stirring, covered, for another 10 minutes, or until the beans and peas are warmed through. Remove from the heat.

3 Season with salt and pepper to taste. Arrange the red pepper strips and olives evenly across the top. Cover and let the paella stand for 5 minutes. Garnish with lemon wedges and parsley, then serve.

2 tbsp olive oil

1 onion, chopped

3 garlic cloves, finely chopped

pinch of saffron threads

pinch of crushed dried chillies

225g (8oz) chopped tomatoes

1 tsp smoked paprika

450g (1lb) uncooked paella rice, such as Bomba or Calisparra

750ml (1¼ pints) vegetable stock

175g (6oz) cooked haricot beans

115g (4oz) cooked pigeon peas or black-eyed beans

125g (4½oz) cooked kidney beans

60g (2oz) frozen green peas, thawed

60g (2oz) jarred roasted red pepper, drained and cut in strips

60g (2oz) pitted, sliced green Spanish olives

1 large lemon, cut into 8 wedges

flat-leaf parsley, to garnish

Make it with fish

Add 225g (8oz) cooked, peeled, prawns along with the red pepper strips in step 3.

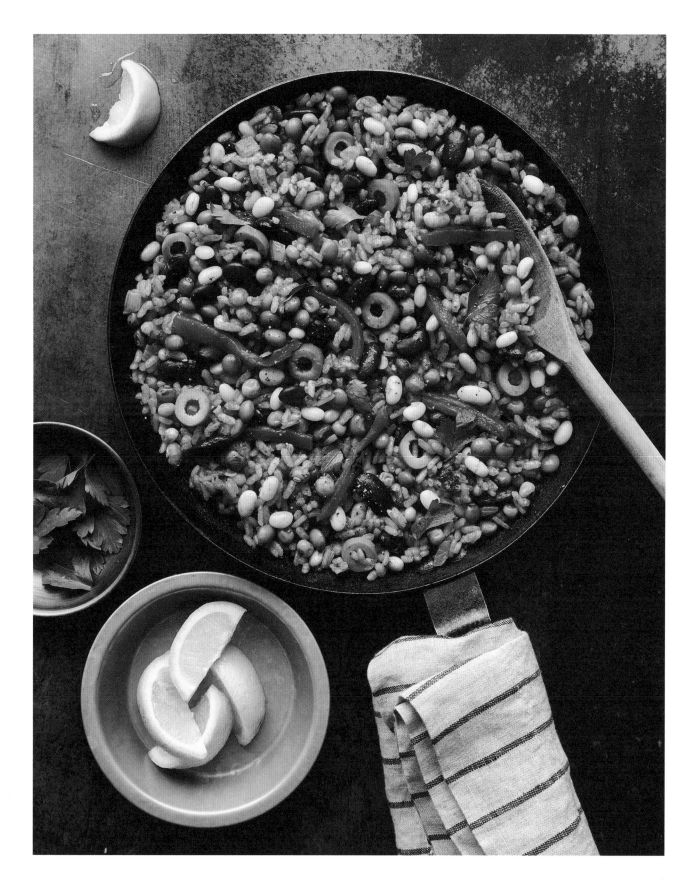

Egyptian Rice

This is a fragrant mix of storecupboard staples – rice and lentils. Dukkah is an Egyptian mix of spices, roasted nuts, and ground sesame seeds. Add toasted almonds or hazelnuts, if you wish.

serves 4   **prep** 15 mins   **cook** 1 hr 15 mins

1 Put the lentils and bay leaf in a heavy-based pan and pour over the stock. Season with salt and pepper, then bring to the boil, reduce the heat to a simmer, cover with the lid, and cook for about 20 minutes (depending on the packet's instructions). Remove the lid and cook for a further 10 minutes or so until the lentils are beginning to soften. Turn off the heat, put the lid back on, and set aside.

2 Put the rice in a separate pan, cover with water so it just skims the top of the rice, and bring to the boil. Reduce to a simmer and cook gently, partially covered with the lid, for about 10 minutes or until the rice is cooked through – you may need to top up the hot water if the rice is becoming dry. Turn off the heat, cover with the lid, and set aside – the rice will continue to steam.

3 Heat the oil in a large flameproof casserole over a medium heat, add the onions, and cook for 8–10 minutes until they just begin to crisp slightly. Add seasoning, stir though the garlic, cumin, and dukkah spice (if using), if using, and cook for a minute. Drain the lentils, then add to the rice, stirring well so all the grains and lentils are coated and everything is heated through. Add the lemon juice and most of the herbs, remembering to remove the bay leaf. Serve topped with the feta or spoon over a tomato-based sauce or plain yogurt. Sprinkle over the remaining fresh herbs to garnish.

200g (7oz) Puy lentils, rinsed and picked over for any stones

1 bay leaf

900ml (1½ pints) hot vegetable stock

salt and freshly ground black pepper

200g (7oz) easy-cook basmati rice

2 tbsp olive oil

2 large onions, sliced

3 garlic cloves, grated

1 tsp cumin

3 tsp Dukkah spice (optional)

juice of 1 lemon

small handful of flat-leaf parsley, finely chopped

small handful of mint leaves, finely chopped

small handful of coriander, finely chopped

200g (7oz) feta cheese, crumbled

Make it vegan

Replace the feta cheese with nut cheese (see page 37).

Vegetable Biryani

In this dish, the rice is cooked first and then is gently steamed in the spiced vegetable mixture. Adjust the vegetable list to suit your refrigerator, adding more or less varieties as you wish.

serves 6 **prep** 30 mins **cook** 1 hr 15 mins

1 Preheat the oven to 180°C (350°F/Gas 4). In a pan of simmering water, cook the rice for 10 minutes or until just tender. Drain and set aside. Cook the carrot and potatoes in a pan of boiling water for about 5 minutes until almost tender. Then add the cauliflower and cook for a further 6–8 minutes until all the vegetables are tender. Drain and set aside.

2 Heat the oil in a large heavy-bottomed pan over a medium heat, add the onion, and cook for 4–5 minutes until soft. Add the red and green peppers and the courgette, and cook for 5 minutes, stirring occasionally. Add the boiled vegetables and frozen peas, then stir in the turmeric, chilli powder, coriander, curry paste, and cumin seeds. Cook for a further 5 minutes, then stir in the stock.

3 Spoon half the rice into an ovenproof dish and top with the vegetable mixture. Top with the remaining rice, cover with foil, and bake for about 30 minutes until hot. Scatter over the cashews and serve with naan, mango chutney, lime pickle, or raita.

350g (12oz) basmati rice

1 large carrot, peeled and sliced

2 potatoes, peeled and chopped into small pieces

½ cauliflower, chopped into small florets

3 tbsp vegetable oil

1 red onion, chopped

1 red pepper, deseeded and chopped

1 green pepper, deseeded and chopped

1 courgette, chopped

85g (3oz) frozen peas

1 tsp ground turmeric

1 tsp mild chilli powder

2 tsp ground coriander

2 tsp mild curry paste

1 tsp cumin seeds

150ml (5fl oz) hot vegetable stock

60g (2oz) cashew nuts, lightly toasted

Make it with meat

Add 500g (1lb 2oz) cubed chicken thigh fillets to the pan after the onions in step 2. Stir over the heat for 5 minutes and then continue as per the recipe.

Roasted Vegetable Farro Risotto

This rich and delicious risotto uses farro for its chewy texture and slightly sweet flavour. The addition of roasted vegetables makes this a warm and satisfying meal.

serves 4   **prep** 15 mins   **cook** 40 mins

1 Preheat the oven to 200°C (400°F/Gas 6). Heat 1 tablespoon of the oil in a large saucepan over a medium heat. Add the onion and cook for about 5 minutes, stirring frequently, until softened. Then add the farro, stir to mix, and cook gently for 1-2 minutes.

2 Stir the wine into the pan and leave to cook until all the liquid has been absorbed. Then add the stock a ladleful at a time, stirring constantly, allowing the liquid to be fully absorbed before adding more. Once all the liquid has been absorbed, add the Parmesan and thyme, and season to taste. Remove from the heat.

3 Meanwhile, arrange the red peppers, courgette, and tomatoes in a baking tray. Drizzle over the remaining oil and season with salt and pepper. Transfer the tray to the oven and roast the vegetables for 20-25 minutes, stirring occasionally, until cooked through and golden. Stir the roasted vegetables into the risotto and serve immediately.

3 tbsp light olive oil

1 small onion, finely chopped

150g (5½oz) uncooked farro

120ml (4fl oz) white wine

1 litre (1¾ pints) hot vegetable stock

50g (1¾oz) freshly grated Parmesan cheese

1 tbsp finely chopped thyme

sea salt and freshly ground black pepper

1 red pepper, deseeded and thinly sliced

1 courgette, diced

150g (5½oz) cherry tomatoes

Make it with fish

Stir in 500g (1lb 2oz) cooked, peeled prawns to the risotto with the roasted vegetables in step 3.

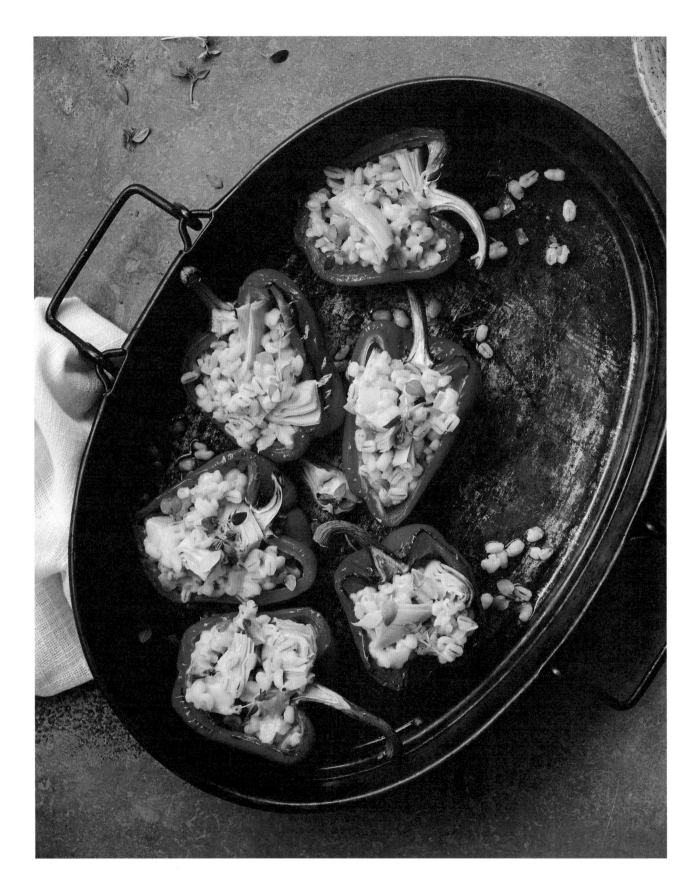

Red Peppers Stuffed with Artichoke Barley Risotto

These lightly roasted sweet red peppers are the perfect vessels for a creamy barley risotto dotted with artichoke hearts and are a delightful change from the conventional stuffed peppers.

serves 6 **prep** 10 mins **cook** 35 mins

1 Heat 2 tablespoons of the oil in a large saucepan over a medium heat. Add the onion and cook, stirring frequently, for 5–10 minutes or until translucent and lightly browned. Then add the barley, stir to mix, and cook for a further 1–2 minutes.

2 Stir the wine into the pan and leave to cook until all the liquid has been absorbed. Then add the stock a ladleful at a time, stirring constantly, allowing the liquid to be fully absorbed before adding more. Once all the stock has been added, cook, stirring constantly, for a further 2–3 minutes or until all the liquid has been absorbed. Remove from the heat, stir in the Parmesan and artichoke hearts, and season to taste.

3 Preheat the oven to 180°C (350°F/Gas 4). Slice the red peppers in half lengthways. Then, core, deseed, and remove the white ribs from the inside and discard. Rub the peppers with the remaining oil and place on a baking sheet lined with foil. Roast in the oven for 15 minutes, until softened. Remove from the heat. Divide the risotto mixture into 6 equal parts and use to fill the peppers. Serve immediately.

4 tbsp extra virgin olive oil

1 small onion, diced

225g (8oz) uncooked barley

125ml (4¼fl oz) white wine

1 litre (1¾ pints) warm vegetable stock

100g (3½oz) freshly grated Parmesan cheese

350g (12oz) artichoke hearts, chopped

salt and freshly ground black pepper

6 red peppers

Make it vegan

Simply omit the Parmesan cheese or replace is with a plant-based Parmesan or nut cheese (see page 37).

Cauliflower Hazelnut Polenta

It may seem fiddly to skin the hazelnuts, but the skins can be quite bitter and will change the taste of the dish if left on. The sweetness of the roasted nuts contrasts well with the cauliflower and the ripeness of the Manchego.

serves 4   **prep** 15 mins   **cook** 55 mins

1 Preheat the oven to 180°C (350°F/Gas 4). Spread the hazelnuts out on a baking sheet, place in the oven, and toast for 10–15 minutes or until they are well browned with the skins peeling off. Leave them to cool slightly. Then place them between two pieces of kitchen paper and rub to remove the skins. Roughly chop the hazelnuts and set aside.

2 Increase the heat to 200°C (400°F/Gas 6). Place the cauliflower on a large baking sheet, drizzle over the oil, and season well. Place in the oven and roast for 30 minutes, stirring occasionally, until golden brown and cooked through. Remove from the heat, drizzle over the lemon juice, and set aside.

3 For the polenta, place the milk and 500ml (16fl oz) of water in a large, lidded saucepan. Add ¼ teaspoon salt and a good grinding of pepper. Bring to the boil, then reduce the heat to medium-low. Gradually add one-third of the polenta, stirring constantly, until well combined. Then add the remaining polenta, stirring constantly, and cook for about 10 minutes or until it is well combined and smooth.

4 Reduce the heat to low and cover partially. Cook for a further 15 minutes, stirring occasionally to ensure it does not stick to the bottom, until it is creamy. Add a little more water or milk to the pan if the polenta seems too thick. Then stir in the butter and cheese and mix well to incorporate. Remove from the heat. Spoon the polenta into serving bowls and top with the hazelnuts and cauliflower. Garnish with the parsley and serve immediately.

75g (2½oz) hazelnuts

450g (1lb) cauliflower, cut into florets

1 tbsp olive oil

salt and freshly ground black pepper

juice of half a lemon

For the polenta

500ml (16fl oz) milk, plus extra if needed

150g (5½oz) coarse polenta

3 tbsp unsalted butter

30g (1oz) grated Manchego cheese, plus extra to serve

handful of flat-leaf parsley, roughly chopped, to garnish

Why not try...

Instead of Manchego cheese, try using Pecorino Romano. Parmesan will work too, however it has a stronger flavour and saltiness so you might not need as much.

Make it vegan

To make the polenta, bring 1 litre (1¾ pints) vegetable stock to the boil in a large, lidded saucepan. Add the polenta and cook according to steps 3 and 4. When the polenta is smooth and thick stir in 60ml (2fl oz) soy milk, 3 tbsp nutritional yeast and 1–2 tbsp plant-based butter.

Desserts

Desserts and sweet treats can still be enjoyed on a flexitarian diet. These recipes include plenty of vegan variations too, making them perfect for when you are reducing your intake of animal products.

Strawberry Polenta Shortcakes

These little "sandwiches" are a lovely adaptation of the traditional shortcake. They make excellent use of polenta to produce the perfect dessert for summer, when you can take advantage of a glut of strawberries.

serves 6 **prep** 30 mins **cook** 40 mins

1 Preheat the oven to 190°C (375°F/Gas 5). Line two baking trays with greaseproof paper and set aside. Place 1 litre (1¾ pints) of water in a large saucepan and bring to a simmer. Then add the polenta and cook for 2–3 minutes, stirring constantly, until it has thickened. Remove from the heat and leave to cool for about 2 minutes.

2 Add the oil, sugar, and vanilla extract and mix well. Divide the mixture equally between the two baking trays, spreading it out to a 5mm (¼in) thick layer. Place the trays in the oven and bake for 30 minutes or until the polenta is spongy and slightly firm to the touch. It should easily pull away from the paper. Remove from the heat and leave to cool.

3 Place the cooled polenta on a clean work surface and use a cookie cutter to cut out twelve 8cm (3in) wide rounds. Place the double cream in a large bowl and whisk until it is thick and holds its shape. Place one-third of the strawberries in a bowl and crush with the back of a fork. Add half the icing sugar and mix well to combine. Cut the remaining strawberries into thin slices.

4 To assemble the shortcakes, lay one polenta round on each of six plates. Top them with 1 tablespoon of the whipped cream, 1 tablespoon of the strawberry and sugar mixture, and a few slices of strawberries. Place the remaining polenta rounds on top and gently pat them dry with kitchen paper. Dust with icing sugar and serve immediately.

200g (7oz) polenta
2 tbsp light olive oil
40g (1½oz) sugar
1 tsp vanilla extract
300ml (10fl oz) double cream
500g (1lb 2oz) strawberries
20g (¾oz) icing sugar

Make it vegan

Refrigerate a 400ml can coconut milk overnight and remove the thick, solid milk at the top of the can into a bowl. Using an electric mixer, beat the coconut milk on medium-high until smooth. Add 2 tbsp icing sugar and continue beating until the milk is fluffy and resembles whipped cream. Use this in place of the whipped double cream in step 4.

Sweet Spiced Freekeh with Fresh Figs

Inspired by the cuisine of the Middle East, in this dish the freekeh is cooked with sweet spices to enhance its flavour and served with honey, pistachios, and figs for an aromatic and mouth-watering dessert.

serves 4　**prep** 5 mins　**cook** 25 mins

1　Place the freekeh, star anise, cardamom, cinnamon, ginger, and nutmeg in a large saucepan. Add the salt and cover with 500ml (16fl oz) of water. Place the pan over a medium heat and bring to the boil. Then reduce the heat to a simmer and cook for about 15 minutes or until all the liquid has been absorbed.

2　Meanwhile, preheat the grill to its medium setting. Grease and line a baking tray with greaseproof paper. Cut a cross in the top of each fig, cutting almost to the bottom so they open up like a flower. Place on the baking sheet and drizzle with 2 tablespoons of honey. Place the tray under the grill and cook for 10 minutes or until the figs are lightly grilled.

3　Remove and discard the star anise and cardamom pods. Add the remaining honey to the cooked freekeh and mix well. Divide the freekeh mixture between four plates. Top each plate with two grilled figs and a quarter of the pistachios. Garnish with mint and drizzle with honey, if you wish. Serve with Greek yogurt.

100g (3½oz) cracked freekeh

1 star anise

4 cardamom pods

1 tsp ground cinnamon

½ tsp grated fresh root ginger

¼ tsp grated nutmeg

¼ tsp salt

8 fresh figs, stems removed

4 tbsp honey, plus extra to serve

40g (1½oz) pistachios, roughly chopped

2 tbsp chopped mint leaves

4 tbsp Greek yogurt, to serve

Why not try...

In place of the freekeh, you can use the same quantity of polenta.

Make it vegan

Replace the honey with agave nectar and the Greek yogurt with coconut yogurt (see page 38).

Almond Polenta Cake with Raspberries

This gluten-free cake is perfect for satisfying your sweet tooth while staying away from flour. The polenta and almonds give the cake a crumbly texture that beautifully offsets the tartness of the raspberries.

serves 8-10   **prep** 15 mins, plus cooling   **cook** 45 mins

1 Preheat the oven to 180°C (350°F/Gas 4). Grease and line a 23cm (9in) springform cake tin with greaseproof paper. Cream the butter and sugar with an electric whisk for 2 minutes or until light and fluffy. Add the eggs one at a time, mixing well between additions. Then add the almond extract and whisk for 2 minutes until fully incorporated.

2 Place the ground almonds, polenta, and baking powder in a separate bowl and mix well. Lightly fold the dry mixture into the butter, sugar, and egg mixture until just smooth. Gently fold the raspberries into the batter. Spoon the batter into the prepared tin, smooth over the surface, and scatter over the flaked almonds.

3 Bake the cake for 45 minutes or until golden brown and a skewer inserted into the centre comes out with only a few crumbs. Leave the cake in the tin to cool slightly. Then transfer to a wire rack to cool completely before serving. Store in the fridge, in an airtight container, for up to 3 days.

200g (7oz) unsalted butter

230g (8oz) unrefined caster sugar

3 large eggs

1 tsp almond extract

200g (7oz) ground almonds

100g (3½oz) polenta

1½ tsp baking powder

200g (7oz) raspberries

20g (¾oz) flaked almonds

Make it vegan

Instead of unsalted butter, use the same amount of vegetable oil spread. Whisk together 3 tbsp flax seeds with 9 tbsp warm water and let is stand for 15 minutes. Use this mixture in place of the eggs in step 1.

Chocolate Chip, Peanut, and Buckwheat Cookies

Gluten-free buckwheat flour adds to the nuttiness of these delicious cookies. Perfect for children and adults alike, enjoy them with a cup of tea or your morning coffee.

makes 12 large cookies   **prep** 30 minutes, plus chilling and cooling   **cook** 15 minutes

1 Line two baking sheets with greaseproof paper and set aside. In a large bowl, cream together the butter and sugar with an electric whisk until light and fluffy. Then beat the egg into the mixture until well combined.

2 Place the flour, salt, and baking powder in a separate bowl and mix well. Fold the dry mixture into the butter, sugar, and egg mixture, a little at a time, until thoroughly incorporated. Add the chocolate chips and peanuts to the mixture and stir well to incorporate. Cover the dough with cling film and chill in the fridge for about 30 minutes. Preheat the oven to 180°C (350°F/Gas 4).

3 Place golf ball-sized pieces of the dough on the prepared baking sheets and flatten them gently. Make sure they are placed at least 5cm (2in) apart, as they will spread while baking. Bake the cookies for about 15 minutes, until they start to turn golden but still look a little underbaked. Remove from the heat and leave on the baking sheet for at least 10 minutes to cool and firm up. Then transfer to a wire rack to cool completely. Store in an airtight container.

110g (4oz) unsalted butter

175g (6oz) brown sugar

1 large egg

200g (7oz) buckwheat flour

¼ tsp salt

½ tsp baking powder

85g (3oz) dark chocolate chips

85g (3oz) salted peanuts

Make it vegan

Replace the unsalted butter with the same amount of vegetable oil spread. Mix 1 tbsp flax seeds with 3 tbsp warm water and let is sit for 15 minutes. Add this mixture instead of the egg in step 1. Most dark chocolate is vegan, but check the label to be sure.

Apple and Cinnamon Crumble

This is a beloved dessert, and deservedly so. A good crumble topping should be loosely patted down over the filling, and made with irregular-sized lumps of butter that melt and create a fudge-like texture during the bake.

serves 6-8   **prep** 25 mins   **cook** 45 mins

1   Preheat the oven to 180°C (350°F/Gas 4). Combine the flour, sugar, and cinnamon in a large bowl. Rub in the butter until the mixture resembles coarse breadcrumbs, making sure you leave a few small lumps of butter.

2   For the filling, place the apple pieces in the ovenproof dish. Scatter over the sugar, flour, and cinnamon. Toss well to combine. Gently pack the filling into the dish.

3   Dot the filling with butter, then spoon the flour topping over and spread it out gently. Lightly shake the dish to help settle the topping into an even layer.

4   Bake for 45 minutes, until the top is golden brown and the filling is soft when pierced with a sharp knife. Remove and leave to rest for 5 minutes. Serve warm with cream, if desired. You can store the crumble, covered in the fridge, for up to 3 days.

250g (9oz) plain flour

150g (5½oz) caster sugar

1 tsp cinnamon

150g (5½oz) unsalted butter, softened and diced

For the filling

8-10 dessert apples, peeled, cored, and diced into 2cm (¾in) pieces

2 heaped tbsp soft light brown sugar

1 heaped tbsp plain flour

½ tsp ground cinnamon

25g (scant 1oz) butter, softened and diced

double cream, to serve (optional)

23cm (9in) ovenproof dish, about 7.5cm (3in) deep

Make it vegan

Use an equal amount of vegetable oil spread in place of the unsalted butter.

Plum and Thyme Galette

Fold over the pastry edges to make this free-form tart – this process helps to contain the juices of the sweet, sticky plums. You could also replace the plum with another orchard fruit.

serves 6-8   **prep** 20 mins, plus chilling and cooling   **cook** 40 mins

1 Sift the flour and sugar into a large bowl and mix well. Rub in the butter until the mixture resembles fine breadcrumbs. Add the salt and 3 tablespoons of ice-cold water to the bowl.

2 Use your fingertips to bring the mixture together to form a dough, adding more cold water if needed. Transfer the dough to a lightly floured surface and knead it gently and briefly until smooth. Wrap it in cling film and chill for at least 1 hour.

3 Preheat the oven to 200°C (400°F/Gas 6). On a lightly floured surface, roll out the pastry to a 30cm (12in) round. Transfer it to a large baking sheet sprinkled with a little water.

4 For the filling, combine the almonds and 1 tablespoon of the sugar in a bowl. Sprinkle it over the pastry, leaving a 5cm (2in) border.

5 Arrange the plum slices over the filling in a spiral pattern. Fold the pastry edges over them, pressing down lightly to enclose the filling. Brush the pastry edges with the milk, sprinkle the plums with the remaining sugar, and place the thyme in the centre.

6 Bake in the oven for 35–40 minutes, until the plums are soft and the pastry is golden. Remove from the heat and leave to cool for 10 minutes. Then remove the thyme and serve warm with single cream, if using.

225g (8oz) plain flour, plus extra for dusting

25g (scant 1oz) caster sugar

125g (4½oz) unsalted butter, chilled and diced

pinch of salt

1 tbsp milk

3 sprigs of thyme

single cream, to serve (optional)

For the filling

1 tbsp ground almonds

3 tbsp caster sugar

3 large ripe plums, stoned and thinly sliced

Make it vegan

Replace the unsalted butter with an equal amount of vegetable oil spread, and use soy milk instead of cow's milk.

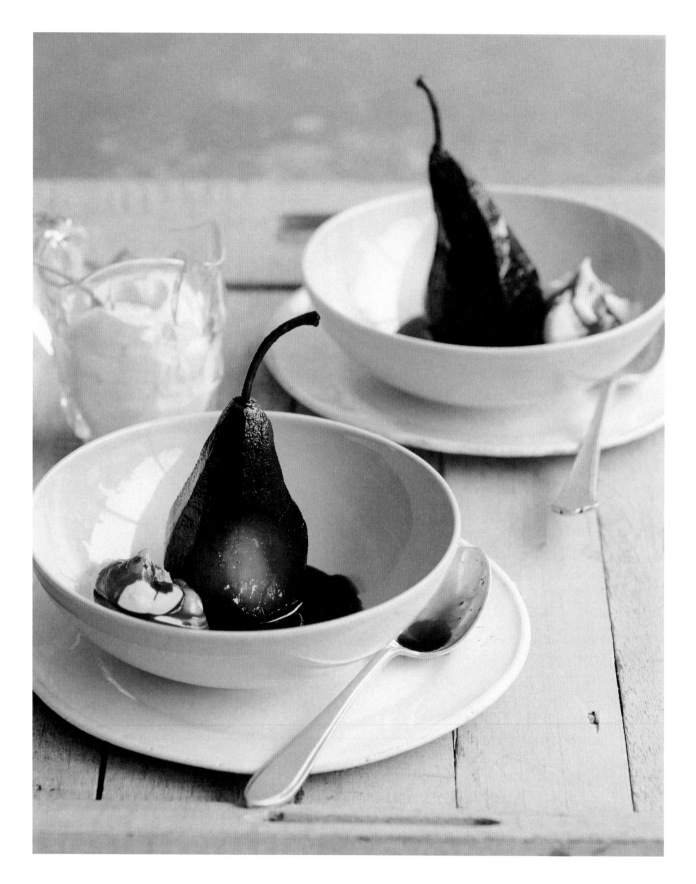

Poached Pears in Red Wine

Taking on the rich purple hues of red wine, poached pears are a simple and classic dessert. Here the pears are laced with cinnamon, orange zest, and a little fresh thyme. The flavours deepen the longer the pears are kept in the cooking liquid.

serves 4   **prep** 10 mins, plus cooling and chilling   **cook** 35–45 mins

1 Place the wine, sugar, cinnamon, orange zest, and thyme in a lidded, heavy-based saucepan. Bring to the boil, stirring until the sugar melts. Then reduce the heat to a low simmer.

2 Slice a disc off the base of each pear to allow it to stand upright. Add them to the pan, making sure they are submerged in the wine. Cover and cook for 20–30 minutes, until the pears are just soft when pierced with a knife.

3 Remove and cool to room temperature. Transfer the pears and cooking liquid to a large dish and cover with cling film. Chill until needed, or overnight to darken the colour. Bring to room temperature before serving. Then discard the cinnamon, orange zest, and thyme.

4 Strain 200ml (7fl oz) of the cooking liquid into a heavy-based saucepan. Bring to the boil, then reduce the heat to a simmer. Cook for 15 minutes, until slightly thickened. Leave to cool until just warm. Place the pears upright on serving plates and pour over a little of the sauce. Serve warm with whipped cream, if using.

750ml (1¼ pints) red wine

150g (5½oz) caster sugar

1 cinnamon stick

peeled zest of 1 orange

1 sprig of thyme

4 just-ripe pears, peeled

whipped cream, to serve (optional)

Triple Chocolate Chip Brownies

The best kind of brownie is crisp on the surface and gently yielding on the inside. If you prefer them really soft and gooey, bake them for 5 minutes less than suggested here. If you like them firm, add 5 minutes more to the cooking time.

makes 9   **prep** 20 mins, plus cooling   **cook** 50 mins

1 Preheat the oven to 180°C (350°F/Gas 4). Lightly grease and line a 20cm (8in) square cake tin with baking parchment, leaving some overhang. Melt the butter and both lots of chocolate in a heatproof bowl over a saucepan of simmering water, making sure it does not touch the water. Stir until smooth, then leave to cool.

2 Gradually add the vanilla extract and both lots of sugar to the mixture and whisk well to combine. Then add the eggs, one at a time, whisking well after each addition until smooth. Place the flour, cocoa powder, salt, and baking powder in a separate bowl and mix well.

3 Use a spatula to fold the dry ingredients into the chocolate mixture and combine until smooth. Then mix in both lots of chocolate chips until evenly incorporated. Pour the brownie mixture into the prepared tin, and spread it out evenly.

4 Bake for 40–45 minutes, until an inserted toothpick comes out clean. Leave to cool slightly before removing the brownie from the tin. Then cut it into nine equal-sized pieces, cleaning the knife with a damp kitchen towel between cuts. Serve warm with vanilla ice cream, if desired. You can store them in an airtight container for up to 5 days.

115g (4oz) unsalted butter, plus extra for greasing

175g (6oz) good-quality dark chocolate, finely chopped

60g (2oz) very dark chocolate, at least 85 per cent cocoa solids, finely chopped

2 tsp vanilla extract

200g (7oz) caster sugar

50g (1¾oz) dark brown sugar

2 large eggs

125g (4½oz) plain flour

3 tbsp natural cocoa powder

¾ tsp salt

¼ tsp baking powder

60g (2oz) good-quality milk chocolate chips

60g (2oz) white chocolate chips

vanilla ice cream, to serve (optional)

Make it vegan

Replace the unsalted butter with the same amount of vegetable oil spread. Mix 2 tbsp flax seeds with 6 tbsp warm water. Let it sit for 15 minutes and use the mixture in place of the eggs in step 2. For the chocolate and chocolate chips, choose vegan varieties.

Index

Acknowledgments

DK would like to thank:
DK Australia would like to thank: Lucy Gwendoline Taylor for writing and editing the first chapter of the Australian edition; Sunil Sharma, Pushpak Tyagi, Vikas Sachdeva and Anurag Trivedi from DK India for the internal design; Ella Egidy for the cover design; Niki Foreman for proofreading; and Max McMaster for the index. DK UK would like to thank: Oreolu Grillo and Millie Andrew for editorial assistance, and Nicola Powling for designing the chapter openers.

Text credits
Recipe material in this publication was previously published in *Step by Step Desserts* (2015), *Grains as Mains* (2015), *Healthy Gut Cookbook* (2016), *Modern Australian Vegan* (2018), *Pasta Reinvented* (2018), *Plant-based Cookbook* (2016), *Power Pulses* (2017), *Ramen Noodle Cookbook* (2015), *Sprouted!* (2017) and *The Slow Cook Book* (2018).

Image credits
All images © Dorling Kindersley
For further information see: **dkimages.com**

About the contributor
Lucy Gwendoline Taylor is a Melbourne-based Accredited Practising Dietitian and Accredited Nutritionist with a special interest in whole food, plant-based diets. Alongside her private practice, Lucy maintains a popular blog (BloomNutritionist. com), which features evidence-based, plant-based nutrition information. She has also written about plant-based diets for online and print media publications, including *The Age* and *The Sydney Morning Herald*. She has been vegan since 2013, and aligns with the vegan philosophy for ethical, environmental, and health reasons.

Penguin Random House

Producer Samantha Cross
Producer, pre-production David Almond
Pre-production manager Sunil Sharma
Art editor Vikas Sachdeva
Senior DTP designer Pushpak Tyagi
DTP designer Anurag Trivedi
Jacket designer Ella Egidy
Senior editor Bethany Patch
Editor Paige Farrell
Contributor Lucy Gwendoline Taylor

DK UK
Editor Amy Slack
Senior art editor Glenda Fisher
Jacket designer Nicola Powling
Producer, pre-production David Almond
Producer Samantha Cross
Managing editor Stephanie Farrow
Managing art editor Christine Kielty
Art director Maxine Pedliham
Publisher Mary-Clare Jerram

First British edition, 2019
Dorling Kindersley Limited
80 Strand, London, WC2R 0RL

First Australian edition published in 2019 by DK Australia,
an imprint of Penguin Random House Australia Pty Ltd
707 Collins St, Melbourne, Victoria 3000

Copyright © 2019 Dorling Kindersley Limited
10 9 8 7 6 5 4 3 2 1
001–317109–Dec/2019

All rights reserved.
No part of this publication may be reproduced, stored in or introduced into a retrieval system, or transmitted, in any form, or by any means (electronic, mechanical, photocopying, recording, or otherwise), without the prior written permission of the copyright owner.

ISBN: 978-0-2414-1976-2

Printed and bound in China

A WORLD OF IDEAS:
SEE ALL THERE IS TO KNOW

www.dk.com